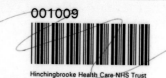
Assessment of Mental Capacity: Guidance for doctors and lawyers

withdrawn 05/24

Second edition

Assessment of Mental Capacity: Guidance for doctors and lawyers

Second edition

This report outlines the current legal requirements in England and Wales concerning assessment of mental capacity. Practical guidelines on the medical assessment of capacity are included.

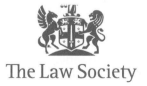
The Law Society

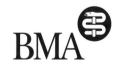
BMA

First published in 1995
Second impression 1997
Third impression 2001
by British Medical Association

Second edition published in 2004
by BMJ Books, BMA House, Tavistock Square,
London WC1H 9JR

www.bmjbooks.com

British Library Cataloguing in Publication Data

A catalogue record for this book is available from the British Library

ISBN 0 7279 1671 8

Typeset by SIVA Math Setters, Chennai, India
Printed and bound in Spain by GraphyCems, Navarra

Contents

Acknowledgements

Contributing authors (second edition, 2004)

Gordon Ashton	Solicitor, District Judge, Deputy Master of the Court of Protection, Preston Combined Court, member of Equal Treatment Advisory Committee of the Judicial Studies Board
Penny Letts	Policy Consultant, Mental Health Act Commissioner, former Law Society Policy Advisor on Mental Health and Disability
Peter Rowlands	Barrister
Edward Solomons	Deputy Official Solicitor and Deputy Public Trustee
Jonathan Waite	Consultant Psychiatrist, Queen's Medical Centre, Nottingham, Lord Chancellor's Medical Visitor

Managing editor	Penny Letts
Editorial staff	Veronica English (BMA)
	Jenny McCabe (Law Society)
	Gillian Romano-Critchley (BMA)
	Ann Sommerville (BMA)

Thanks are due to Denzil Lush, Anthony Harbour and members of the BMA's Medical Ethics Committee and the Law Society's Mental Health and Disability Committee for commenting on earlier drafts.

Contributing authors (first edition, 1995)
Nigel Eastman
Michael Hinchliffe
Penny Letts
Denzil Lush
Steven Luttrell
Lydia Sinclair
Ann Sommerville

Membership of the Working Party for the first edition (1993–1995)

James Birley	Psychiatrist, former BMA President
Nigel Eastman	Forensic psychiatrist and barrister (non-practising). Secretary of the Mental Health Subcommittee of the Royal College of Psychiatrists and member of the Law Society Mental Health & Disability Committee
J Stuart Horner	Chairman, BMA's Medical Ethics Committee
Penny Letts	Secretary, Law Society Mental Health & Disability Committee
Denzil Lush	Solicitor, member of the Law Society Mental Health & Disability Committee
Lydia Sinclair	Solicitor, member of the Law Society Mental Health & Disability Committee, Mental Health Act Commissioner
Ann Sommerville	BMA Advisor on Medical Ethics
David Watts	General practitioner and member of the BMA's Medical Ethics Committee

List of cases

Page numbers are shown in **bold**

List of statutes

Page numbers are shown in **bold**

List of statutory instruments

Page numbers are shown in **bold**

Part I
Introduction

Chapter 1 identifies the key elements in defining what is meant by capacity, and sets these in the context of proposals for reform of incapacity legislation. It describes the background leading to the need for guidance for doctors and lawyers on the assessment of capacity, and explains how this book should be used.

Chapter 2 discusses some key professional and ethical issues for both doctors and lawyers and sets the scene for good practice in the assessment of mental capacity.

1 The law, practice, and this book

1.1 What is capacity?

Capacity is the ability to do something. In a legal context it refers to a person's ability to do something, including making a decision, which may have legal consequences for that person, or for other people.[1] Capacity is the pivotal issue in balancing the right to autonomy in decision making and the right to protection from harm.

The prime principle which underpins both current law and medical practice with regard to issues of mental capacity is, as the Law Commission for England and Wales (the Law Commission) has stated, that people should be "enabled and encouraged to take for themselves those decisions which they are able to take".[2] Doctors and lawyers have common responsibilities to ensure the protection of people who are incapable of deciding matters for themselves and to promote the choices of those who can and should regulate their own lives. The careful assessment of whether individuals have or lack capacity is essential to the protection of their rights. Effective communication, both between the professionals involved and with the person being assessed, is vital. This book sets out to aid communication between doctors and lawyers and clarify the framework within which assessment of capacity takes place.

1.2 The need to define capacity

As advance directives and proxy decision making attract media and public attention, general practitioners and lawyers are increasingly consulted by healthy competent people wishing to make provision for their future care and medical treatment when capacity may be lost. In this and many other areas, doctors and lawyers are frequently asked to define the notion of capacity and explain the test of capacity that might apply, to ensure that the rights and needs of patients and clients are properly recognised.

Capacity, however, can mean something different to each profession, and the manner in which it is assessed can also vary. Although capacity is a legal concept, it is not (at the time of writing) clearly defined in legislation (see section 1.3). The law adopts a functional approach – that capacity must be assessed in relation to the particular decision an individual purports to make at the time the decision needs to be made. The legal capacity (understanding) required for each decision depends on the complexity of the information relevant to the decision and the particular legal test of capacity (if one exists) to be applied. The guidance in this book is intended to help doctors and lawyers reach a common understanding of the requirements of the law in all areas where an assessment of capacity may be needed. It is important that both professions work within their own areas of professional expertise but cooperate with each other in the interests of their clients.

1.3 Proposals for law reform

This book is being published at a time when changes are expected in several areas of legislation affecting people with mental disabilities. It has long been recognised that the law relating to mental incapacity is fragmented, complex, and out of date. Reform of the law in this area has taken a long time to achieve but there are now indications that progress is being made.

In the early 1990s, the Law Commission carried out lengthy and detailed consultations on the adequacy of the law affecting mentally incapacitated adults. In 1995 it published a wide-ranging report recommending a major overhaul of the law.[3] The main recommendation was that there should be a new comprehensive statutory jurisdiction, defining what it means to lack capacity, and setting a framework within which decisions about an incapacitated person's welfare, medical care and property and affairs can be authorised. After some delay and further consultation,[4] the government responded by issuing a policy statement, setting out the proposed changes accepted by the government and announcing its intention to introduce legislation "when Parliamentary time allows".[5]

At the time of writing, no date has been set for this much needed reform, but in December 2002 the Lord Chancellor's Department announced the start of work to prepare draft legislation. Law reform is therefore possible during the lifetime of this book, as a result of which many of the legal provisions discussed would change. Implementation of any new legislation is likely to be staged and will take some time. The implications of proposed reform of the law are mentioned as appropriate throughout this book. Lawyers need to inform themselves immediately when changes in the law are introduced. Doctors will be kept informed of the implications for medical practice through the BMA website (http://www. bma.org.uk/ethics).

As well as an overhaul of the law relating to decision making on behalf of incapacitated adults, other changes in the pipeline include reform of mental health law (not specifically covered in this book but closely linked; see section 1.5.2) and law on sex offences aimed at providing greater protection to vulnerable people (see Chapter 11).

1.3.1 Evolving case law

In one respect the current law is clear and will remain so – all adults are presumed to have legal capacity unless there is evidence to the contrary (see Part II). Similarly, much of the relevant case law (law made by judges in delivering judgments in court cases) described in this book is well established, and will continue to apply, even after new legislation is introduced. Of course, this case law is constantly evolving and will continue to develop as judges refine the interpretation of legal provisions.

In the absence of statute, both professionals and the courts have turned to the Law Commission's report for guidance on the approach to adopt in defining and assessing mental capacity. In particular, the definitions proposed by the Law Commission to ascertain whether a person lacks capacity have found their way into case law and established practice.[6] The government has agreed that the definitions set out below are helpful and are likely to be incorporated in some form in future legislation.[7]

- A person is without capacity if, at the time that a decision needs to be taken, he or she is unable by reason of mental disability to make a decision on the matter in question; or unable to communicate a decision on that matter because he or she is unconscious or for any other reason.
- Mental disability is any disability or disorder of the mind or brain, whether permanent or temporary, which results in an impairment of mental functioning.
- A person is to be regarded as unable to make a decision by reason of mental disability if the disability is such that, at the time the decision needs to be made, the person is unable to understand or retain the information relevant to the decision, or unable to make a decision based on that information.

These definitions reflect the current legal position of a functional test of capacity. Although this has been the position for some time there are, however, indications that in some areas of practice assessments of capacity fall far short of meeting these accepted criteria.[8] It is hoped that the guidance in this book will be helpful in improving practice.

1.4 How to use this book

This book sets out to provide a useful resource tool for both the health and legal professions in England and Wales. It is intended to be a source of key references appropriate to any assessment of mental capacity. Some repetition in the text is unavoidable and is indeed desirable – since it is expected that health and legal professionals will dip into the sections as they are relevant to a particular client rather than read the book from cover to cover. Cross references are indicated where appropriate.

Part II discusses some relevant legal principles as they apply to mental capacity. It provides a general background by explaining the role of the law in relation to assessment of capacity. This material will be familiar to lawyers but may be useful in setting the scene for other professionals.

Part III examines the legal tests of capacity which apply to various decisions or activities an individual may wish to undertake, such as writing a will or getting married. In order for any person to be judged mentally capable of validly undertaking a particular action, he or she must meet legal standards set by statute or by the courts. Different requirements apply to different decisions. Lawyers often seek medical opinions when they are requested to advise or act on behalf of a client whose mental capacity is in doubt. Lawyers who ask doctors to assess a person's capacity should always make clear the activity in which the person intends to engage, or the decision that the person expects to make, and the law's requirements in this respect. Part III, by clarifying the legal requirements for a number of activities or decisions, is primarily intended as a reminder to lawyers and to help doctors who have been asked to conduct an assessment of a person's capacity. References to statute and case law are given where appropriate.

In some cases, medical practitioners have to assess an individual's mental capacity not in order to inform others but to clarify whether medical treatment can proceed without the patient's consent. Whether an apparent consent or refusal of treatment is legally valid is discussed in Chapters 12 and 13, which are aimed primarily at health professionals.

Part IV deals with the medical practicalities of assessing capacity. Chapter 14 sets down accepted practice for carrying out assessments of capacity and will be familiar to practitioners who regularly work in the mental health field. It is primarily intended, therefore, to assist health professionals who only occasionally encounter a request for an assessment of capacity to be carried out. Chapter 15 aims to help lawyers direct their requests appropriately and to be aware of the steps involved in a medical assessment.

There are seven appendices covering: case studies (Appendix A); the role of the Official Solicitor (Appendix B); practice notes of the Official Solicitor on medical and welfare decisions for adults who lack capacity (Appendix C) and Appointment in Family Proceedings (Appendix D); certificates of mental capacity (Appendices E and F); and a sample letter of instruction to a doctor being asked to assess capacity (Appendix G).

1.5 Scope of this book

1.5.1 What is covered?

The civil law and medical practice in England and Wales

This book deals with the legal position in England and Wales regarding the rights and treatment of adults (18 years and over) who may or may not lack mental capacity; it indicates the relationship between law and accepted medical practice. The focus is on civil law, that is those areas of law concerning the private rights of citizens. Reference is included to case law through which the law is constantly evolving. Where relevant, pointers are given to any recommendations for new legislation which are under active consideration by the government (see also section 1.3). Generally, however, the law examined here is that in force at the time of writing (September 2003).

Guidance for doctors and lawyers

The book brings together guidance for doctors and lawyers on what is understood by the concept of capacity in various situations and the role of both professions in the assessment of capacity. Pointers are given for good practice in the assessment of mental capacity. Case studies are provided in Appendix A. The purpose of these examples is to give solicitors and doctors practical guidance:

1 on situations in which it may be necessary to assess a person's capacity
2 on how to assess capacity
3 highlighting any professional or ethical dilemmas that may arise.

Some key professional and ethical issues are discussed further in Chapter 2.

1.5.2 What is not covered?

Children

The book is concerned only with the position of adults. The legal position of children and young people under 18 years is different and is beyond the scope of this book. The BMA has published separate guidance for doctors on all aspects of health care for children and young people.[9] The Law Society has a panel of solicitors assessed as competent to represent children. Details are available at http://www.solicitors-online. com.

Jurisdictions outside England and Wales

The book deals only with the law in England and Wales. It does not deal with other parts of the UK. In Scotland, statutory guidance has been published on the Adults with Incapacity (Scotland) Act 2000, which introduced a new statutory framework for decision making for people with impaired capacity.[10] The BMA has issued separate guidance for doctors on the requirements in Scotland for the assessment of capacity and the treatment of adults who lack capacity to consent.[11]

The criminal law

The book sets out the legal provisions relating only to the civil law, that is those areas of law concerning the private rights of citizens. It does not cover aspects of the criminal law except for one specific area – Chapter 11 deals with the provisions in the criminal law relating to protection of vulnerable people from sexual abuse, which may arise in the context of consent to sexual relationships. Issues such as a defendant's "fitness to plead" or the need for an "appropriate adult" to be present during police questioning are not considered. The Law Society publishes separate guidance for lawyers on advising and representing mentally disordered people who are the subject of criminal investigation or proceedings.[12]

Physical incapacity

This book also does not consider issues arising from a person's physical incapacity. It is recognised that, in some circumstances, it may not be easy to differentiate between physical and mental incapacity, for example when considering the fitness to drive of a person with dementia. Another example is where severe physical disabilities affect a person's ability to communicate wishes or decisions. Every effort should be made to assist people to communicate, but where this is not possible, the same considerations in assessing their capacity will apply as to those with mental disabilities.

Mental health legislation

Even in relation to private rights under the civil law, no consideration is given to those aspects of mental health legislation which relate to detention in hospital or capacity to consent to treatment for mental disorder. Where mental health legislation applies to a patient, its provisions override the provisions of the common law relating to capacity to consent to treatment. Mental health legislation, which was under review at the time of writing, requires professionals to have regard for a code of practice[13] which provides further guidance on how the law should be applied.

There are, however, important interfaces between the common law relating to capacity to consent to medical treatment and the provisions of the Mental Health Act 1983 (in force at the time of writing) which should be made clear.[14] The provisions of the 1983 Act are concerned solely with treatment for mental disorder; it is therefore not possible to use those provisions in order to undertake any surgical or other medical procedures which are unrelated to the patient's mental disorder, no matter how mentally or legally incapacitated the patient may be.[15] At times this interface can be somewhat complex. There may be a question as to whether a particular proposed treatment is "for" the patient's mental disorder. For example, is tube-feeding of a patient with anorexia nervosa regarded as treatment for the patient's mental illness or treatment for its consequences? The courts have decided that a broad view should be taken so that treatment for mental disorder includes treatment for its consequences. This means that some detained patients who have capacity to refuse feeding can nevertheless be treated against their will for physical conditions (such as extreme weight loss) if the physical condition is a consequence of their mental disorder.[16] Where a patient lacks capacity to consent by reason of mental disorder, tube-feeding may be justified under the 1983 Act as above or alternatively in the patient's best interests.[17]

1.6 Where to obtain further advice

Assessing, advising or treating people with impaired capacity are complex matters, often giving rise to professional or ethical dilemmas in both medical and legal practice. Some key issues affecting both professions are discussed in Chapter 2, but further advice may be needed when considering individual cases. Both the British Medical Association and the Law Society offer ethical guidance to their members. Doctors can contact the Ethics Department of the BMA and lawyers the Professional Ethics Division of the Law Society. In addition, advice is also available from bodies such as the Office of the Official Solicitor (see Appendix B) and the Public Guardianship Office (see section 4.2.1). The addresses of these and other organisations are given on pages 221–5.

The Lord Chancellor's Department has issued general guidance on the current legal position on mental incapacity in the form of a series of leaflets for professionals (legal practitioners, healthcare professionals and social care professionals) and for members of the public (people with learning difficulties, relatives and carers of people who lack capacity, and those who wish to plan for future incapacity).[18] These leaflets also include signposts to sources of further guidance and information and provide contact details and website addresses of relevant organisations.

References and notes

1 This description of the meaning of capacity has been adapted from one devised by Denzil Lush, Master of the Court of Protection. Lush D. Legal capacity. In: Whitehouse C, ed. *Finance and law for the older client*. London: LexisNexis Butterworths Tolley, 2000.
2 Law Commission. *Mental incapacity*. London: HMSO, 1995: paragraph 2.46 (Law Com No 231).
3 Ibid. The report includes a draft Mental Incapacity Bill (pp 213–84).
4 Lord Chancellor's Department. *Who decides? Making decisions on behalf of mentally incapacitated adults*. London: HMSO, 1997 (Cm 3803).
5 Lord Chancellor's Department. *Making decisions: the government's proposals for making decisions on behalf of mentally incapacitated adults*. London: The Stationery Office, 1999: paragraph 7 (Cm 4465).
6 See for example: Re C (Adult: Refusal of Medical Treatment) [1994] 1 All ER 819; Re MB (Medical Treatment) [1997] 2 FLR 426.
7 Lord Chancellor's Department. *Making decisions: the government's proposals for making decisions on behalf of mentally incapacitated adults*. Op cit: paragraph 1.6.

8   See for example: Suto WMI, Clare ICH, Holland AJ. Substitute financial decision-making in England and Wales: a study of the Court of Protection. *J Social Welf Fam Law* 2002;**24**:37–54.

9   British Medical Association. *Consent, rights and choices in health care for children and young people.* London: BMJ Books, 2001.

10   The Scottish Executive has published five codes of practice, training materials, public information leaflets and other guidance to assist with the implementation and operation of the Adults with Incapacity (Scotland) Act 2000. See http://www.scotland.gov.uk/justice/incapacity (accessed 24 June 2003).

11   British Medical Association. *Medical treatment for adults with incapacity: guidance on ethical and medico-legal issues in Scotland.* London: BMA, 2002.

12   Postgate D, Taylor C. *Advising mentally disordered offenders.* London: The Law Society, 2000.

13   Department of Health, Welsh Office. *Mental Health Act 1983: code of practice.* London: The Stationery Office, 1999.

14   See for example: R v Bournewood Community and Mental Health NHS Trust ex parte L [1998] 3 All ER 289. For a description of this case see section 12.2. In June 2002, the government issued for consultation a draft Mental Health Bill which proposed additional statutory safeguards for compliant incapacitated patients receiving treatment for mental disorder: Department of Health. *Draft Mental Health Bill.* London: The Stationery Office, 2002: Part 5 (Cm 5538-I).

15   St George's Healthcare NHS Trust v S, R v Collins and others, ex parte S [1998] 3 All ER 673.

16   B v Croydon District Health Authority [1995] 2 WLR 294.

17   R v Collins and Ashworth Hospital Authority ex parte Brady [2001] 58 BMLR 173.

18   Lord Chancellor's Department. *Making decisions: helping people who have difficulty deciding for themselves.* London: LCD, 2003.

2 Professional and ethical issues

2.1 Capacity to instruct a solicitor

In carrying out legal transactions or conducting litigation on behalf of clients with capacity, lawyers must act on their clients' instructions.[1] They have a duty to advise their clients of the legal consequences of the action they are proposing to take, and clients may change their instructions as a result of receiving legal advice. Ultimately, as long as the client has capacity to give instructions, the lawyer must act on those instructions, or cease to act directly on the client's behalf. A key question for lawyers, therefore, is whether the client has capacity to give instructions.

There is a legal presumption of capacity unless the contrary is shown. Solicitors would be acting negligently, however, if they acted on their client's instructions without first satisfying themselves that the client has the requisite level of capacity. Different levels of capacity are required for different transactions; for example very different considerations apply to making a will than to conducting personal injury litigation. A solicitor must therefore assess the client's understanding in the context of the relevant legal test of capacity (as set out in Part III) and then consider whether the client is able to convey in general terms what he or she wants the solicitor to do.

This does not mean that the client must be able to understand all the details of the law – it is the role of the lawyer to provide legal advice. It is also possible that the client may be clear about some aspects of a legal transaction or proceedings, while lacking capacity to deal with others. The Court of Appeal has stressed "the issue-specific nature" of the test of capacity, describing the process as follows:

> ... the requirement to consider the question of capacity in relation to the particular transaction (its nature and complexity) in respect of which the decisions as to capacity fall to be made. It is not difficult

to envisage claimants in personal injury actions with capacity to deal with all matters and take all "lay client" decisions related to their actions up to and including a decision whether or not to settle, but lacking capacity to decide (even with advice) how to administer a large award.[2]

In the same way, lawyers must consider the client's capacity to give instructions in respect of each particular transaction at the time a decision needs to be made. If there is doubt about a client's capacity, it is advisable for the lawyer to seek a medical opinion. It will be necessary to explain to the doctor the relevant legal test of capacity and ask for an opinion as to how the client's medical condition may affect his or her ability to meet the specified legal requirements. The final decision, however, as to whether the client has specific capacity to instruct, rests with the solicitor.

If the solicitor considers that a client lacks capacity to give instructions, the solicitor should generally decline to act on the client's behalf.[3] The client should not, however, be left "high and dry" and action should be taken to protect the client's immediate interests.[4] Depending on the circumstances of the case, special procedures may be used to enable a solicitor to act on behalf of an incapacitated client, for example to put in place safeguards to protect the client's financial affairs (see Chapter 4) or by acting through a receiver, attorney or litigation friend (see Chapter 7) or the Official Solicitor (see Appendix B).

2.2 Confidentiality

Carrying out an assessment of capacity requires doctors and lawyers to share information about the personal circumstances of the person being assessed. Yet doctors, lawyers, and other professionals are bound by a duty of confidentiality towards their clients, imposed through their professional ethical codes and reinforced by law.[5] As a general principle, personal information may only be disclosed with the client's consent, even to close relatives or "next of kin". There are, however, circumstances when disclosure is necessary in the absence of consent:

The decided cases very clearly establish: (i) that the law recognises an important public interest in maintaining professional duties of confidence; but (ii) that the law treats such duties not as absolute but as liable to be overridden where there is held to be a stronger public interest in disclosure.[6]

In relation to people who lack capacity to decide about disclosure, a balance must be struck between the public and private interests in maintaining confidentiality and the public and private interests in permitting, and occasionally requiring, disclosure for certain purposes. Some guidance has been offered in the case of *R (on the application of S) v Plymouth City Council* which concerned an application for disclosure of social services' records to the mother (and nearest relative) of a young adult with learning disabilities, who was subject to a local authority guardianship order under the Mental Health Act 1983. In allowing limited disclosure to the mother, Lady Justice Hale said:

[The young adult's] interest in protecting the confidentiality of personal information about himself must not be underestimated. It is all too easy for professionals and parents to regard children and incapacitated adults as having no independent interests of their own: as objects rather than subjects. But we are not concerned here with the publication of information to the whole wide world. There is a clear distinction between disclosure to the media with a view to publication to all and sundry and disclosure in confidence to those with a proper interest in having the information in question.[7]

A similar balancing act must be carried out by professionals seeking or undertaking assessments of capacity. It is essential that information concerning the person being assessed, which is directly relevant to the decision in question, is made available, to ensure that an accurate and focused assessment can take place. Every effort must first be made to obtain the person's consent to disclosure by providing a full explanation as to why this is necessary and the risks and consequences involved. If the person is unable to consent or refuse, relevant disclosure – that is the minimum necessary to achieve the objective of assessing capacity – may be permitted where this is in the person's interests. This does not mean, however, that everyone has to know everything. Specific guidance for lawyers and doctors is given in the following sections.

2.2.1 Lawyers

There is a general principle that "a solicitor is under a duty to keep confidential to his or her firm the affairs of clients and to ensure that the staff do the same".[8] This general duty is qualified by an exception which states that "express consent by a client to disclosure of information relating to his or her affairs overrides any duty of confidentiality".[9] Although "the duty to keep a client's confidences can be overridden in certain exceptional circumstances"[10] there is no specific exception which permits informing a doctor about the contents of a client's will, or the extent of his or her property and affairs, without first having obtained express consent from the client.

There have been decisions however in cases involving wills, in which such disclosure may appear to be authorised. In *Kenward v Adams* the judge stated that there is a "golden if tactless rule" that "when a solicitor is drawing up a will for an aged testator or one who has been seriously ill, it should be witnessed and approved by a medical practitioner, who ought to record his examination of the testator and his findings ... [and] that if there was an earlier will it should be examined and any proposed alterations should be discussed with the testator"[11] (see sections 3.5 and 5.4). Any solicitor who cannot obtain from his or her client consent to the disclosure of confidential information should seek advice from the Professional Ethics Division of the Law Society.

2.2.2 Doctors

Doctors are bound by a professional duty to maintain the confidentiality of personal health information unless the patient gives valid consent to disclosure or, if the patient is incapable of giving consent, the doctor believes disclosure to be in that person's best interests. Difficult decisions may arise if relatives, carers or the patient's lawyer approach the doctor for a medical report on an individual whose capacity to understand and consent is in doubt, but the patient refuses to be assessed (this is discussed further in section 2.4) or else agrees to assessment but not to disclosure of the results. The statutory body for doctors, the General Medical Council, recognises that there are some exceptional circumstances when disclosure of confidential information can be made in an incapacitated patient's interest without consent (see section 12.6). More detailed ethical guidance on confidentiality and disclosure of health information, which draws together guidance from professional and regulatory bodies, is available from the BMA.[12]

2.3 Creating the right environment for assessing capacity

Where there are doubts about capacity, it is important that people are assessed when they are at their highest level of functioning because this is the only realistic way of determining what they may or may not be capable of doing. It may be helpful to consult a relative or someone close to the person being assessed to consider how this may be achieved, so long as this does not compromise the person's right to confidentiality (see section 2.2).

Detailed guidance on the practical aspects of assessing capacity is given in Part IV. The following pointers may be helpful to both doctors and lawyers to create the right environment and to optimise the conditions for assessing capacity.[13]

- Try to minimise anxiety or stress by making the person feel at ease.
- If the cause of the incapacity can be treated, the doctor should treat it before the assessment of capacity is made.
- If the person's capacity is likely to improve, wait until it has improved. Obviously, if the assessment is urgent it may not be possible to wait.
- Be aware of any medication which could affect capacity (for example medication which causes drowsiness). Consider delaying the assessment until any negative effects of medication have subsided.
- If there are communication or language problems, consider enlisting the services of a speech therapist or an interpreter, or consult family members on the best methods of communication.
- Be aware of any cultural, ethnic or religious factors which may have a bearing on the person's way of thinking, behaviour or communication.

- Choose the best time of day for the examination. Some people are better in the morning; others are more alert in the afternoon or early evening.
- Be thorough, but keep the assessment within manageable time limits to avoid tiring or confusing the client.
- Avoid obtrusive time-checking. It should be possible, without too much discernible eye movement, to keep a check on the time.
- If more than one test of capacity has to be applied, try to do each assessment on a different day if possible.
- Choose the best location. Usually people feel more comfortable in their own home than in a doctor's surgery or a lawyer's office.
- Try and ensure that there are no obstructions which could hinder the development of a relationship of equals: for example, the height and positioning of the chairs.
- As far as possible make sure that the temperature in the room is comfortable and that the lighting is soft and indirect, but sufficiently bright for easy eye contact and interpretation of expression, and to study any relevant documentation.
- Consider whether or not a third party should be present. In some cases the presence of a relative or friend could reduce anxiety; in others their presence might actually increase anxiety. In some cases a third party might be a useful interpreter, but in others this could be intrusive.
- Try and eliminate any background noise or distractions, such as the television, the radio, or people talking.
- If possible make sure that assessments cannot be overheard or interrupted, including, for example, a telephone.
- Be sensitive towards other disabilities, such as impaired hearing or eyesight, which could appear to inhibit the person's capacity, but which, with appropriate aids, could be overcome.
- Speak at the right volume and speed. Try to use short sentences with familiar words. If necessary, accompany speech with slightly exaggerated gestures or facial expressions and other means of non-verbal communication.
- If necessary, provide verbal or visual aids to stimulate and improve the person's memory.

- If carrying out more than one test of cognitive functioning, allow a reasonable time for general relaxed conversation between each test to avoid any sense of disappointment at failing a particular test.
- Try to avoid subjecting the client to an increasingly demoralising sequence of "I don't know" answers.

2.4 Refusal to be assessed

There may be circumstances in which a person whose capacity is in doubt refuses to undergo an assessment of capacity, or refuses to be examined by a doctor. It is usually possible to persuade someone to agree to an assessment if the consequences of refusal are carefully explained. For example, it should be explained to people wishing to make a will (see Chapter 5) that the will could be challenged and held to be invalid after their death, while evidence of their capacity to make a will would prevent this from happening. Similarly, an enduring power of attorney (see section 4.1) could be challenged without evidence of the donor's capacity, with the result that the attorney chosen by the donor may be unable to act. Further, it may not be possible to pursue legal proceedings unless the court is satisfied that a party to the proceedings has capacity (see Chapter 7). It should perhaps also be explained that the solicitor may have to decline to act on the person's behalf if there are doubts about the person's capacity to give instructions (see section 2.1).

If the client is unable to consent to or refuse assessment, it will normally be possible for an assessment to proceed, so long as the person is compliant and this is considered to be in the person's best interests (see section 2.5). In the face of an outright refusal, however, no one can be forced to undergo an assessment of capacity unless required to do so by a court in legal proceedings. Even then, entry to a person's home cannot be forced, and a refusal to open the door to the doctor may be the end of the matter. Where there are serious concerns about the person's mental health, an assessment under mental health legislation may be warranted as long as the statutory grounds are fulfilled.

2.5 People assessed as lacking capacity

Both lawyers and doctors need to appreciate that if an individual is judged to lack capacity to make the decision in question, any act or decision taken on that person's behalf must be in that person's best interests. The notion of best interests has been current in the common law for some time (see for example Chapters 12 and 13 on capacity to consent to medical procedures).

The Law Commission endorsed the concept of "best interests" and recommended that when deciding what is in a person's best interests consideration should be given to:

- the past and present wishes of the individual
- the need to maximise as much as possible the person's participation in the decision
- the views of others as to the person's wishes and feelings
- the need to adopt the course of action least restrictive of the individual's freedom.[14]

The government accepted these recommendations and proposed two further considerations – the prospects of the person recovering mental capacity and the need to be satisfied that the person's wishes were not formed under undue influence.[15]

In May 2003, the Lord Chancellor's Department published a series of guidance leaflets (see section 1.6) intended to provide help and guidance for adults who – due to mental incapacity – may need support to make decisions, and also for relatives, carers and professionals who may be involved in the decision making process.[16] These leaflets also provide practical suggestions to help in determining what may be in the best interests of a person without capacity.

2.6 Summary of points for doctors

The following is a brief summary of issues about which doctors should be aware in carrying out an assessment of capacity.

- In law, people are presumed to have capacity unless the contrary is shown.
- Capacity should be assessed in relation to the particular decision or activity rather than a general assessment of the patient's condition. Doctors should assess what the person is actually capable of deciding at the time a decision needs to be made, not whether the decision is sensible or wise.
- In many situations where a judgment about legal capacity has to be made a doctor's opinion will be obtained. A GP, consultant, other hospital doctor, prison doctor, or forensic physician may be approached to provide this. If the medical practitioner is not routinely involved in assessing capacity, the practical steps outlined in Part IV may provide a helpful guide. Assessment requires some knowledge of the person, including his or her ethnicity, cultural or religious values and social situation. More than a brief interview and reading of other medical reports is often necessary.
- Capacity, however, is ultimately a legal concept, defined by law (see Part II). The doctor must assess the person's capacity in relation to whatever activity that person is attempting to carry out. The understanding (legal capacity) required for each decision depends on the complexity of the information relevant to the decision and the legal test (if one exists) to be applied. Doctors who are asked to give an assessment of an individual's capacity must be clear about the relevant legal test (see Part III) and should ask a lawyer to explain it, if necessary.
- Every person is entitled to privacy and confidentiality (see section 2.2). If the doctor does not know the person, however, it may be necessary to seek views from others with professional and personal knowledge of the individual and knowledge of the specific decision in question. Assessment of whether a person has capacity to manage their own financial affairs, for example, depends partly on the amount and complexity of the assets involved. A doctor who is asked to provide a medical report in such a case needs some knowledge of the person's assets and the skills required to administer them.
- When asked to assess a person with a learning disability, doctors should not rely solely on prior reports giving an

estimated "mental age" but must ensure that a current assessment is made. Statements of a person's mental age may be misleading if they do not reflect the person's experience and the context for the particular decision. These concerns also apply to people with fluctuating capacity. Assessments of capacity should be regularly reviewed.

- In some circumstances health professionals may be asked to witness a patient's signature on a legal document. By witnessing the document it may be inferred that the doctor or nurse is confirming the patient's capacity to enter into the legal transaction effected by the document, rather than merely indicating that the witness has seen the patient sign the document. Doctors and nurses should be clear as to what they are being asked to do (see section 3.5).

2.7 Summary of points for lawyers

The following is a brief summary of points for lawyers to bear in mind when acting for a person who may lack capacity.

- In carrying out legal transactions or conducting litigation on behalf of clients with capacity, lawyers must act on their clients' instructions. Ultimately, so long as the client has capacity to give instructions, the lawyer must act on those instructions, or cease to act directly on the client's behalf. Before taking action on behalf of a client, the solicitor must be satisfied that the client has the capacity to give instructions in relation to the transaction or decision in question (see section 2.1).
- There is a legal presumption of capacity unless the contrary is shown. Whether a client has capacity is a matter of law, to be determined by applying the correct legal test. Different levels of capacity are required for different activities. If there is doubt about a client's mental capacity, it is advisable for the lawyer to seek a medical opinion. Medical practitioners should be asked to give an opinion as to the client's capacity in relation to the particular activity or action in question, rather than a general assessment of the client's mental condition. In order to do this, the lawyer has a responsibility to explain to the doctor the

relevant legal test of capacity (see Part III). It should not be assumed that doctors automatically understand what is being asked of them.

- It is important to choose a doctor who has the skills and experience to carry out the particular assessment. This may be the person's GP in situations where familiarity with and personal knowledge of the patient may be helpful. In some cases, a specialist with expertise in the patient's particular medical condition may be preferable. Chapter 15 provides further guidance.

- Doctors' assessments assume more weight in borderline cases or in those at risk of challenge, which together form the majority of cases upon which doctors and lawyers need to liaise. The most obvious cases of incapacity, such as when a person is unconscious or has very severe learning disabilities, are less likely to require detailed medical confirmation. Similarly, where the person is demonstrably capable of dealing with the matter in hand, medical assessment is superfluous. Fluctuating capacity presents particular difficulties – medical evidence is likely to be essential to demonstrate a person's capacity to take action during a lucid interval (see section 3.2.2).

- Capacity can be enhanced by the way explanations are given, by the timing of them or by other simple measures discussed in this book. It can be impaired by fatigue, pain, anxiety, or unfamiliar surroundings. Yet doctors are constantly working under constraints of time or location and other limitations, including perhaps their own preconceptions or prior reports from other people about the extent of the individual's capacity. Doctors are also trained with the concept of promoting the patient's interests in all circumstances. It is therefore important to ask doctors to assess what the person is actually capable of deciding at the time a decision needs to be made, not whether the decision is sensible or wise.

References and notes

1 The Law Society. *The guide to the professional conduct of solicitors, 8th ed.* London: The Law Society, 1999: paragraph 12.08.
2 Masterman-Lister v Brutton & Co and Jewell & Home Counties Dairies [2003] 3 All ER 162:173.

3   The Law Society. *The guide to the professional conduct of solicitors, 8th ed*. Op cit: paragraph 12.12. An exception is the representation of patients before the Mental Health Review Tribunal. See: The Law Society Mental Health and Disability Committee. *Representation at mental health review tribunals: guidelines for legal representatives*. London: The Law Society, 1998.

4   The Law Society. *The guide to the professional conduct of solicitors, 8th ed*. Op cit: paragraph 24.04; note 2.

5   Convention for the protection of human rights and fundamental freedoms: Article 8. (4. ix. 1950; TS 71; Cmnd 8969) Data Protection Act 1998.

6   W v Egdell and others [1990] 1 All ER 835:848.

7   R (on the application of S) v Plymouth City Council [2002] 1 WLR 2583: 2599.

8   The Law Society. *The guide to the professional conduct of solicitors, 8th ed*. Op cit: paragraph 16.01.

9   Ibid: paragraph 16.02; note 2.

10 Ibid: paragraph 16.02.

11 Kenward v Adams (1975) The Times, 29 November 1975.

12 British Medical Association. *Confidentiality and disclosure of health information*. London: BMA, 1999.

13 This list was devised by Denzil Lush, Master of the Court of Protection. Lush D. Legal Capacity. In: Whitehouse C, ed. *Finance and law for the older client*. London: LexisNexis Butterworths Tolley, 2000.

14 Law Commission. *Mental incapacity*. London: HMSO, 1995: paragraph 3.28 (Law Com No 231).

15 Lord Chancellor's Department. *Making decisions: the government's proposals for making decisions on behalf of mentally incapacitated adults*. London: The Stationery Office, 1999: paragraph 1.12 (Cm 4465).

16 Lord Chancellor's Department. *Making decisions: helping people who have difficulty deciding for themselves*. London: LCD, 2003.

Part II
Legal principles

Part II discusses some relevant legal principles as they apply to mental capacity.

Chapter 3 provides a general background by explaining the role of the law and the relevance of different types of evidence in relation to assessment of capacity. This material will be familiar to lawyers but may be useful in setting the scene for other professionals. Suggestions are made for both doctors and lawyers about ways of putting these principles into practice. Specific guidance is given to doctors who are asked to witness legal documents.

3 What are the legal principles?

3.1 Capacity and the role of the courts

Whether an individual has or lacks capacity to do something is ultimately a question for a court to answer. It is not a decision that can be made conclusively by the family; or the proprietor of a residential care home; or a social worker; or a solicitor; or even a doctor – although their opinions as to capacity may be of assistance in enabling a court to arrive at its conclusions.[1] Capacity is ultimately a question for the courts because people with an interest in the outcome may wish to challenge an assessment, either on their own behalf or on behalf of the person who is alleged to lack capacity.

In practice, of course, doctors, solicitors, social workers and carers make this sort of decision every day of the week, and very few cases ever get as far as a court. Nevertheless, the courts are keen to safeguard their overall jurisdiction in these matters.[2] By making a decision on capacity, anyone with authority over an individual can deprive that person of civil rights and liberties enjoyed by most adults and safeguarded by the Human Rights Act 1998.[3] Alternatively, such a decision could permit the person lacking capacity to do something, or carry on doing something, whereby serious prejudice could result to either the person lacking capacity or to others. Doctors and lawyers should always bear this in mind: if they conclude someone has or lacks capacity to enter into a transaction they might have to justify to a court their reasons for that conclusion. It is, therefore, helpful to know what effect an opinion could have on the individual concerned. For example, it could restrict, protect, or empower them.

If a case goes to court, the judge has to:

1 decide what the facts are
2 apply the law to those facts
3 come to a decision.

Others involved in making decisions about capacity might find it useful to follow the same steps.

3.2 Capacity and the law of evidence

3.2.1 Presumptions

To keep any investigation of the facts within manageable bounds, courts apply various rules of evidence. These are based on conclusions (presumptions) which must, or may, be drawn from particular facts. Presumptions are either irrebuttable or rebuttable. If a presumption is irrebuttable, it is not open to challenge and the court *must* arrive at a particular conclusion, regardless of any evidence to the contrary. If a presumption is rebuttable, the court has to assume that certain facts are true until the contrary is proved. The most well known rebuttable presumption is the presumption of innocence: anyone charged with a criminal offence is presumed to be innocent until proved to be guilty.

Two important rebuttable presumptions apply to mental capacity.

- The presumption of competence. An adult is presumed to be competent, or to have the mental capacity to enter into a particular transaction, until the contrary is proved. The burden of proof rests on those asserting incapacity (see section 3.2.3).
- The presumption of continuance. Once it has been proved that someone is incompetent, or lacks capacity, this state of affairs is generally presumed to continue until the contrary is proved.

The Court of Appeal has held, however, that where there is evidence that a person has become incapable as a result of a head injury sustained in an accident, the presumption of continuance cannot always be relied on.[4] This is because the person may recover after treatment and should not automatically be deprived of rights because of an initial period of incapacity. In these cases, the burden of proof remains on whoever asserts incapacity (see section 3.2.3).

3.2.2 Lucid intervals

The presumptions of competence and continuance tend to suggest that a person is either constantly capable or constantly incapable. Competence can fluctuate, however, and an intermittent state of capacity is known at law as a "lucid interval". Generally speaking, a deed or document signed by someone who lacks capacity is void and of no effect. But if it is signed during a lucid interval it may be valid. This will almost certainly need to be confirmed by medical evidence (see section 3.2.6).

3.2.3 The burden of proof

Generally, if someone alleges something, that person has to prove it. In cases involving mental capacity the burden of proof is affected by the operation of the presumptions of competence and continuance. So the burden of proof is on the person who alleges that:

- someone lacks capacity (because capacity is presumed until the contrary is proved)
- someone who previously lacked capacity has now recovered and is capable (because incapacity is presumed to continue until the contrary is proved); this does not apply immediately in personal injury cases, however, since the person may recover capacity after treatment, and in such cases, the burden of proof remains on those asserting incapacity (see section 3.2.1)
- something was validly done by an otherwise incapacitated person during a lucid interval (also because of the presumption of continuance).

The case of *Re Sabatini*[5] illustrates the operation of these rules (this case is discussed in more detail in section 5.6). When Mrs Ruth Sabatini was 90 and suffering from Alzheimer's disease, she destroyed a will she had made 25 years earlier, which left her estate to her favourite nephew. If she had had capacity her action would have revoked or cancelled the will, and the nephew would have lost his inheritance. Because of the presumption of competence the judge had to presume that Mrs Sabatini had the capacity to revoke the will unless the contrary was proved by acceptable evidence. The burden of proof, therefore, fell on the nephew to prove to the court that his aunt lacked capacity to revoke the will and that the earlier will made in his favour remained in effect. As it turned out, he was able to produce compelling medical evidence of her incapacity at the time she destroyed the will.

3.2.4 The standard of proof

Those on whom the burden of proof rests must prove their case to a particular standard. There are two standards of proof: "beyond reasonable doubt" which only applies in criminal proceedings; and "the balance of probabilities" which applies in civil proceedings. In deciding whether or not someone has capacity to enter into a particular transaction or make a particular decision, the standard of proof is the civil standard – the balance of probabilities. In practical terms this is the most important rule of evidence in assessing capacity. Having decided what the facts are, and having applied the law to those facts, the assessor must then decide whether the individual is more likely to have capacity, or more likely to lack capacity to do something.

3.2.5 Character evidence and similar fact evidence

As a general rule in both civil and criminal cases, judges will not admit in evidence any information about a person's character or similar events to those now under consideration which have happened in the past. The reason for this rule is that this sort of evidence, although relevant, could be prejudicial and so it is regarded as inadmissible and is not taken into account by the judge (although the government has put forward proposals which could lead to the removal or weakening of this rule in criminal cases). In civil cases, however, a person's psychiatric history is usually highly relevant to the question of capacity and is therefore almost always admissible.

The court may also take into account other witness or documentary evidence which is relevant to the person's capacity to take the decision in question. For example, in the *Masterman-Lister* case (see section 4.2.4) the court gave detailed consideration to Mr Masterman-Lister's diaries, letters and computer documents.[6] The court must however be "alive to the fact that [it is] ... investigating ... capacity not outcomes, although of course outcomes can often cast a flood of light on capacity".[7]

3.2.6 Opinion evidence and expert evidence

In court proceedings witnesses are usually confined to stating the facts, what they have seen or heard, and are not permitted to express their own opinion. An exception is made in the case of expert witnesses who are entitled not only to say what they have seen and heard but also to express the opinion they formed as a result. There is no formal definition as to what constitutes expertise. In general, people will be treated as experts if they have devoted time and attention to the particular branch of knowledge involved, or if they have had practical experience of it and, in some cases, if they have acquired a reputation for being skilled in it.

Whether or not it is justifiable, the law tends to regard any registered medical practitioner as a *de facto* expert on mental capacity, and therefore considers them entitled to express an opinion as to whether a person is or was capable of understanding the nature and effects of a particular transaction. The Court of Appeal has confirmed that in almost every case where a court is required to make a decision as to capacity, it needs medical evidence to guide it,[8] although this will not necessarily be given greater weight than other relevant evidence (see section 3.2.7). Not all doctors do have a sufficient level of knowledge or expertise to determine issues of capacity, however.[9] In giving an opinion on capacity, doctors should set out their qualifications and experience which may have a bearing on their expertise in assessing capacity. The BMA issues guidelines for doctors who are considering acting as expert witnesses.[10]

3.2.7 The weight of evidence

Whether or not the burden of proof is discharged depends on the weight and value which the judge attaches to the various strands of evidence. This involves weighing up the credibility or reliability of the evidence, and ultimately comes down to deciding which version of events is more likely to be correct. Although the courts attach a great deal of weight to medical evidence, one doctor's opinion may not be shared by another, and it is not unprecedented for a judge to favour the evidence of someone who is not even medically qualified. For example, in the case of *Birkin v Wing*[11] the judge preferred the evidence of a solicitor – who considered that the client was mentally capable of entering into a particular contract – to that of a doctor who said that the client lacked capacity.

3.3 Practical suggestions for solicitors instructing doctors

Solicitors asking a doctor to provide medical evidence as to whether or not a client is capable of doing something should do, or bear in mind, the following points.

- It cannot automatically be assumed that all doctors are experts in these matters (see Chapter 15).
- The quality of the doctor's evidence depends heavily on the quality of the instructions he or she is given.
- Be clear about the specific capacity that needs to be assessed, whether it be capacity to enter into a contract; capacity to marry; capacity to create an enduring power of attorney; or capacity to manage and administer one's property and affairs (see Part III).
- Inform the doctor about the legal test to be applied, so if the client proposes to make a will, explain to the doctor the criteria for making a will (see Chapter 5).
- Explain the legal test in simple language that an ordinary intelligent person, who is not a qualified lawyer, can understand (for example, say what is meant by the "nature and effect" of a particular document).
- Let the doctor have all the relevant information needed to reach an informed opinion (for example, if an application is being made to the Court of Protection for the appointment of a receiver, the doctor needs to know something about the client's property and affairs in order to assess whether or not that client is incapable, by reason of mental disorder, of managing and administering such property and affairs) (but see section 2.2 on confidentiality).

- Make sure that the doctor is aware that the standard of proof is the balance of probabilities, rather than beyond reasonable doubt.
- Remind the doctor that his or her opinion on the client's capacity is open to challenge (and as a courtesy the doctor should be informed if the matter is likely to be contentious, without giving the impression that a lower standard of care will suffice in a non-contentious case).
- Wherever possible avoid asking for simultaneous assessments of a client's capacity for a variety of different transactions (for example, where a client is in the early stages of dementia it would be unreasonable to expect the doctor to assess in one examination whether the client is capable of making a will, creating an enduring power of attorney, making a lifetime gift, and managing and administering his or her property and affairs) – not only is this unfair to the doctor, but also could be extremely unfair to the client.

3.4 Practical suggestions for doctors receiving instructions from solicitors

Doctors assessing capacity at the request of a solicitor should bear the following points in mind.

- Guidance for doctors who have limited experience in assessing capacity is given in Chapter 14, but doctors should decline instructions from solicitors if they feel that they have insufficient knowledge or practical experience to make a proper assessment of capacity.
- Solicitors should be asked for more information if necessary. Do not automatically assume that the solicitor is an expert in these matters or has passed on all relevant details.
- If necessary, further information should be asked about:

  - details of the test of capacity that the law requires, with an explanation of that test in simple language that an ordinary intelligent person who is not legally qualified can understand
  - why a medical opinion is being sought and what effect the opinion might have on the patient or client

- the patient's property, affairs and family background if they are relevant to the particular type of capacity to be assessed
- whether the matter is likely to be contentious or disputed (but do not be pressurised into making a decision that will please the solicitor or the patient's family or one faction of the patient's family).

- Wherever possible, keep reports specific, rather than general. Remember that:

  - a laconic opinion lacking detail, diagnosis and reasons is likely to be of little value in terms of evidence
  - the opinion could deprive the individual of a liberty that most adults enjoy
  - the opinion could allow the individual to do something or to carry on doing something which could be extremely prejudicial to the individual or somebody else
  - the opinion could affect the availability of certain financial benefits or services
  - doctors can be called on by a court to give an account of the reasons for arriving at a particular opinion.

3.5 Witnessing documents

Medical professionals, especially those working in hospitals, are often reluctant to witness a patient's signature on a document. This is understandable because, more often than not, the professional status of a doctor or nurse is being invoked in order to lend greater credibility to a transaction. In the section on capacity and the law of evidence (section 3.2.6) a distinction was drawn between ordinary witnesses and expert witnesses. Ordinary witnesses are expected merely to state what they have seen or heard. When it comes to witnessing a signature on a document, an ordinary witness simply states that the document was signed by a person in his or her presence. Expert witnesses are in a different position, because they are invited not only to say what they have seen or heard but also to express an opinion. As was mentioned earlier, the law tends to regard medical practitioners as *de facto* experts on mental capacity. So when a doctor witnesses someone's signature on a document, there is a strong inference that the doctor considered the patient to have the requisite capacity to enter into the transaction effected by the document. If doctors are not confident about the person's capacity, they should decline to act as a witness. They should also decline to act as a witness if they are likely to benefit from it personally.

3.5.1 When medical evidence should be obtained – the "golden rule"

Obtaining medical evidence about a person's capacity is sometimes required by the law (for example, when an application is made to the Court of Protection; see section 4.2), while in other cases, it is merely desirable or a matter of good practice. There are particular circumstances, however, where the law virtually demands that a doctor should witness a person's signature, thereby providing medical evidence as to the person's capacity. For example, in 1975 in *Kenward v Adams*[12] the judge laid down what he called "the golden if tactless rule" that, where a will has been drawn up for an elderly person or for someone who is seriously ill, it should be witnessed or approved by a medical practitioner. The judge assumed that the doctor would not only make a formal assessment of capacity but also record his or her examination and findings. The need to observe this "golden rule" was repeated in 1977 in *Re Simpson*[13] and restated in *Buckenham v Dickinson*[14] (in 1997) in which the solicitor was criticised for failing to follow the "golden rule".

Doctors and nurses therefore need to be clear about what they are being asked to do. It is recommended that, in cases where there is any doubt about a patient's capacity to enter into a particular transaction, doctors and nurses should only witness the patient's signature on a document when:

- they have formally assessed the patient's capacity
- they are satisfied that, on the balance of probabilities, the patient has the requisite capacity to enter into the transaction effected by the document
- they make a formal record of their examination and findings.

Some trusts reportedly prohibit their staff from witnessing legal documents. In such cases, health professionals should take advice from the trust before acting as a witness.

3.5.2 Sample certificate of capacity

We reproduce here a sample form for a certificate of capacity, which may be useful to doctors to record their assessment of a person's capacity in respect of a particular decision or transaction. This may be helpful as a record of the circumstances in which doctors are called upon to witness documents and of their examination and findings.

Sample certificate of capacity

- I (*full name and professional qualifications of medical practitioner*) of (*address*) CERTIFY as follows:
- (*Full name and date of birth of patient*) has been a patient of mine since (*date*) and I have seen him/her (*describe in general terms the degree of regularity, for example approximately four times a year*).
- On (*date*) I examined the patient for the purpose of assessing whether s/he is capable of (*describe the transaction, for example making a will, signing an enduring power of attorney*).
- In my opinion, the patient is not suffering from any mental disability/is suffering from mental disability, namely (*describe the mental disability, for example dementia*).
- In my opinion the patient is capable/incapable of (*describe the transaction as above*).
- I base my opinion on the following grounds: (*state the reasons as fully as possible*).

Signed:
Dated:

References and notes

1   Richmond v Richmond (1914) 111 LT 273. Martin Masterman-Lister v (1) Jewell (2) Home Counties Dairies and Martin Masterman-Lister v Brutton & Co [2002] Lloyds Rep Med 239.
2   See for example: Re MB (Medical Treatment) [1997] 2 FLR 426. R (on the application of Wilkinson) v Broadmoor Special Hospital Authority and

others [2002] 1 WLR 419. Re B (Adult: Refusal of Medical Treatment) [2002] 2 All ER 449. Martin Masterman-Lister v (1) Jewell (2) Home Counties Dairies and Martin Masterman-Lister v Brutton & Co [2002]. Op cit.

3 The Human Rights Act 1998, which came into effect in October 2000, incorporates into UK law the bulk of the substantive rights set out in the European Convention on Human Rights.

4 Masterman-Lister v Brutton & Co and Jewell & Home Counties Dairies [2003] 3 All ER 162. The details of this case are described in section 4.2.4.

5 Re Sabatini (1970) 114 SJ 35.

6 Martin Masterman-Lister v (1) Jewell (2) Home Counties Dairies and Martin Masterman-Lister v Brutton & Co [2002]. Op cit.

7 Masterman-Lister v Brutton & Co and Jewell & Home Counties Dairies [2003]. Op cit: 181.

8 Ibid: 173.

9 Jackson E, Warner J. How much do doctors know about consent and capacity? *J R Soc Med* 2002;**95**:601–3.

10 British Medical Association Medico-legal Committee. *The expert witness: a guidance note for BMA members.* London: BMA, 2001.

11 Birkin v Wing (1890) 63 LT 80.

12 Kenward v Adams (1975) The Times, 29 November 1975.

13 Re Simpson (Deceased), Schaniel v Simpson (1977) 121 SJ 224.

14 Buckenham v Dickinson [1997] CLY 661.

Part III
Legal tests of capacity

Chapters 4–11 examine the legal tests of capacity which apply to various decisions or activities an individual may wish to undertake. Different requirements apply to different decisions. By providing separate clarification of the legal requirements for a number of activities or decisions, each chapter is primarily intended as a reminder to lawyers and to help doctors who have been asked to conduct an assessment of a person's capacity. References to statute and case law are given where appropriate.

In some cases, medical practitioners have to assess an individual's mental capacity not in order to inform others but to clarify whether medical treatment, and sometimes medical research, can proceed without the patient's consent. Capacity to consent and whether an apparent consent or refusal of treatment is legally valid are discussed in Chapters 12 and 13, which are aimed primarily at health professionals.

4 Capacity to deal with financial affairs

4.1 Powers of attorney

A power of attorney is a deed by which one person (the donor) gives another person (the attorney) the authority to act in the donor's name and on his or her behalf in relation to the donor's property and financial affairs. At the time of writing, an attorney has no power to make decisions concerning personal matters or medical care and treatment on behalf of the donor (although this is an area where law reform is proposed; see section 4.1.7).

A power of attorney can be specific or general. If it is specific, the attorney only has the authority to do the things specified by the donor in the power. If it is general, the attorney has the authority to do "anything that the donor can lawfully do by an attorney" in relation to property and financial affairs.[1] The law imposes certain restrictions on what actions a donor can delegate to an attorney. For example, an attorney cannot execute a will on the donor's behalf, nor act in situations which require the personal knowledge of the donor (such as acting as a witness in court). Therefore under a general power of attorney, the attorney only has the authority to do what the donor can lawfully delegate to someone else.

There are two types of powers of attorney; firstly, an ordinary power of attorney which ceases to have effect if the donor becomes mentally incapable; and secondly, an enduring power of attorney which "endures" or continues to operate after the donor has become mentally incapable, provided that it is registered with the Court of Protection (see section 4.2.1).

4.1.1 Ordinary powers of attorney

The test of capacity which a person must satisfy in order to make a power of attorney is that the donor understands the nature and effect of what he or she is doing. An ordinary power of attorney (one which is not "enduring") tends to be used as a temporary expedient: for example, where the donor is going abroad for several months and needs someone to look after various legal or financial transactions during his or her absence. The traditional view is that the capacity required to create an ordinary power of attorney is co-existent with the donor's capacity to do the act which the attorney is authorised to do. If there is any doubt as to the donor's capacity to do the act in question, it would be advisable for the donor to create an enduring power, rather than an ordinary power, so long as the donor has the requisite capacity to do so (see section 4.1.3).

4.1.2 Enduring powers of attorney

Enduring powers of attorney (EPAs) became available in England and Wales in March 1986, when the Enduring Powers of Attorney Act 1985 came into force. The Act itself says nothing about the degree of understanding the donor needs in order to make a valid enduring power – this point was later settled in a court case (see section 4.1.3) – but it does require the power to be in a prescribed form.[2] The form contains most of the basic relevant information that the donor needs to understand, and the procedures to be adopted when executing (signing) an enduring power. The prescribed form is divided into three parts.

- Part A is a page of information explaining what an enduring power is; how the prescribed form should be completed; when and how the power should be registered with the Court of Protection; and informing donors that they can cancel the EPA at any time before it has to be registered. It is essential to the validity of an enduring power that the explanatory notes in Part A are read by or to the donor before he or she signs Part B of the prescribed form.
- Part B contains the actual appointment of the attorney(s), and it should be executed (signed) by the donor in the presence of one witness. A second witness is only necessary if the form is not signed by the donor personally but by someone else in the donor's presence and at the donor's direction (possibly because a physical disability prevents the donor from signing it personally).

- Part C explains some of the duties of an attorney and should be executed by the attorney in the presence of a witness.

Unless the enduring power specifically states that it will not come into force until the donor is mentally incapacitated (which is rare), the power is "live" from the moment the donor executes it. In other words, the attorney can act under it straight away, even though the donor may still be perfectly capable of looking after his or her own property and affairs. If the enduring power is not registered with the Court of Protection, the donor and the attorney have what is known as concurrent authority. Both of them can manage and administer the donor's property and affairs.

An attorney acting under an enduring power must apply to the Court of Protection for the registration of the power if the attorney has reason to believe that the donor is, or is becoming, incapable – by reason of mental disorder – of managing and administering his or her property and affairs.[3]

The donor and his or her closest relatives must be informed of the attorney's intention to register the power. There is a statutory list of relatives in a Schedule to the Enduring Powers of Attorney Act 1985[4] which is similar to, but not the same as the list of nearest relatives in the Mental Health Act 1983. Both the donor and any of the relatives have the right to object to the registration of the power: for example, if they believe that the donor is not yet incapable of managing his or her affairs, or that the power may be invalid, for example because it has been revoked by the donor. Once the power has been registered by the Court of Protection, the donor and the attorney no longer have concurrent authority. Only the attorney has the authority to manage and administer the donor's property and affairs. If, however, even after registration the donor has capacity to perform some tasks, such as running a bank account or shopping, the fact that the power has been registered should not as matter of practice prevent the donor from carrying out these activities.

At the time of writing, the government was looking at what procedural changes could be made to the current system of enduring powers of attorney which could be introduced without primary legislation. Section 4.4 suggests ways in which professional advisers can guard against the risk of financial abuse, particularly at the time of assessing capacity.

4.1.3 Capacity to make an enduring power of attorney

The law states that a power of attorney signed by a person who lacks capacity is null and void, unless it can be proved that it was signed during a lucid interval (see section 3.2.2). Shortly after the Enduring Powers of Attorney Act 1985 came into force the Court of Protection received a considerable number of applications to register enduring powers which had only just been created. This raised a doubt as to whether the donors had been mentally capable when they signed the powers. The problem was resolved in the test case *Re K, Re F*[5] in which the judge discussed the capacity to create an enduring power.

Having stated that the test of capacity to create an enduring power of attorney was that the donor understood the nature and effect of the document, the judge in the case set out four pieces of information which any person creating an EPA should understand:

- if such be the terms of the power, that the attorney will be able to assume complete authority over the donor's affairs
- if such be the terms of the power, that the attorney will be able to do anything with the donor's property which the donor could have done
- that the authority will continue if the donor should be or should become mentally incapable
- that if the donor should be or should become mentally incapable, the power will be irrevocable without confirmation by the Court of Protection.[6]

It is worth noting that the donor need not have the capacity to do all the things which the attorney will be able to do under the power. The donor need only have capacity to create the EPA.

4.1.4 Immediate registration of an enduring power of attorney

The judge in *Re K, Re F* also commented that if the donor is capable of signing an enduring power of attorney, but is incapable of managing and administering his or her own property and affairs, the attorney has an obligation to register the power with the Court of Protection straight away. In a significant number of cases, applications for registration received by the Court of Protection involve enduring powers which have been created less than 3 months before the application was made.[7] Arguably, the attorney also has a moral duty in such cases to forewarn the donor that registration is not merely possible but is intended immediately.

The decision in *Re K, Re F* has been criticised for imposing too simple a test of capacity to create an enduring power. But the simplicity or complexity of the test depends largely on the questions asked by the person assessing the donor's capacity. For example, if the four pieces of basic relevant information described by the judge in *Re K, Re F* were mentioned to the donor, and if the donor was asked "do you understand this?" in such a way as to encourage an affirmative reply, the donor would probably pass the test with flying colours and, indeed, the test would be too simple. If, on the other hand, the assessor were specifically to ask the donor "what will your attorney be able to do?" and "what will happen if you become mentally incapable?" the test would be substantially harder. It can be inferred from the decision in *Re Beaney (deceased)*,[8] confirmed by the Court of Appeal in *Re W (Enduring Power of Attorney)*,[9] that questions susceptible to the answers "yes" or "no" may be inadequate for the purpose of assessing capacity.

Although the legislation does not require the donor's execution of an enduring power of attorney to be witnessed by a doctor, where the donor is of borderline capacity it is advisable that the power be witnessed or approved by a medical practitioner, who should record the findings.[10] Section 3.5 provides guidance for medical practitioners on the procedures to be followed when asked to witness documents. Solicitors instructed to draw up an EPA on behalf of a client must first be satisfied that the client has the required capacity, assisted by a medical opinion where necessary. Further guidance for solicitors on EPAs has been issued by the Law Society.[11]

4.1.5 Registration of an EPA

In signing Part B of the EPA document, the attorney undertakes to register the power with the Court of Protection when the attorney has reason to believe that the donor is or is becoming mentally incapable. The test is that the donor is incapable, by reason of mental disorder, of managing his or her own affairs (see section 4.2). There is no requirement on the attorney to obtain a medical report or otherwise substantiate a "belief" that the donor lacks capacity, but in cases of doubt it may be prudent to obtain confirmation from a doctor to counteract any objection that the donor has not yet become mentally incapable.

Part of the process of applying for registration requires the attorney formally to notify the donor, and at least three close relatives of the donor, that an application has been made, and give them the opportunity to object to the registration. Objections can be made on one or more of the following grounds:[12]

- that the power is not valid as an EPA (for example because the donor lacked capacity at the time of execution of the power or because the document is defective in some way)
- that the power no longer subsists (has become obsolete, for example because it has been cancelled or revoked by the donor (see section 4.1.6) or the attorney is unable or unwilling to act)
- that the application is premature because the donor is not yet mentally incapable
- that fraud or undue pressure was used to induce the donor to make the EPA
- that the attorney is unsuitable to be the donor's attorney.

The burden of proof is on the objector(s) to establish the ground(s) of objection to the satisfaction of the court.[13]

4.1.6 Capacity to revoke a power of attorney

Until an application for registration has been made, the donor may revoke or destroy a power of attorney at any time. If the donor does so, but the attorney believes the donor lacks the capacity to revoke the power, the attorney can apply for registration of the power. The donor may then object to the registration on the ground that the power is no longer valid, and the court must decide whether this ground for objection is established. After registration, no revocation of an enduring power by the donor is valid unless and until the Court of Protection confirms the revocation.

There have been no reported decisions on capacity to revoke an EPA. The evidence which the Court of Protection requires to see in order to be satisfied that the donor has the necessary capacity to revoke the power is as follows[14] whereby the donor should know:

- who the attorney(s) are
- what authority the attorney(s) have
- why it is necessary or expedient to revoke the EPA
- what the foreseeable consequences of revoking the power are.

In practice, where the donor of a registered EPA wishes to revoke it, the attorney often disclaims – that is, gives notice to the Court of Protection – that he or she wishes to cease acting as attorney. The court must then decide whether the donor has capacity to resume management of his or her own affairs, or whether a receivership order or some other order should be made in respect of the donor (see section 4.2).

4.1.7 Proposals for law reform

In its 1995 report the Law Commission recommended the repeal of the Enduring Powers of Attorney Act 1985. In its place the Commission recommended the creation of a new type of power of attorney which would encompass decisions about the donor's personal welfare and medical treatment, as well as the person's property and financial affairs.[15]

The government undertook further consultation,[16] in particular on the safeguards needed to guard against abuse. The government has indicated that it intends to introduce legislation containing provisions about the form and manner of execution of the power, procedural requirements and restrictions on who may be an attorney.[17] In the draft Mental Incapacity Bill published for consultation in June 2003, this was called a "lasting power of attorney" (LPA). The Bill proposes:

- a mandatory prescribed form for an LPA
- a requirement for a certificate as to the capacity of the donor to be signed by a person of a "prescribed description" as set out in regulations

- that where an LPA confers the authority to make decisions about the donor's personal welfare (including giving or refusing consent to medical treatment) the LPA cannot be used unless the donor lacks capacity to give or refuse consent
- that the LPA only permits the attorney to refuse life-sustaining medical treatment where it contains express provision to that effect.

4.2 Capacity to manage property and affairs

If a person who has not made an enduring power of attorney becomes incapable, by reason of mental disorder, of managing and administering his or her property and affairs, it may be necessary for someone to apply to the Court of Protection for an order setting out how the person's affairs may be dealt with, and where necessary for a receiver to be appointed to deal with the day-to-day management of that person's affairs. The powers of the Court of Protection (described in section 4.2.1) are set out in Part VII of the Mental Health Act 1983 (which will continue to remain in force if legislation to amend the compulsory treatment provisions in the 1983 Act is introduced prior to mental incapacity law reform).

The Court of Protection is required to look at medical evidence before it considers appointing a receiver or making any other order concerning the person's affairs. The court's rules specifically state that the evidence must be provided by a registered medical practitioner[18] who is expected to complete a printed medical certificate known as form CP3 (see Appendix F). In consultation with the Royal College of Psychiatrists and the British Medical Association the court has prepared a set of notes which accompany form CP3 and which provide useful guidelines as to the sort of information the court is looking for. Ideally, any doctor who completes a form CP3 should have some knowledge of:

- the Court of Protection
- mental disorder
- the patient

- the patient's property and affairs
- how to assess whether a person is incapable, by reason of mental disorder, of managing and administering his or her property and affairs.

4.2.1 The Court of Protection

The Court of Protection is an office of the Supreme Court, and its function is to oversee the management of the property and affairs of people who are mentally incapable of managing their own affairs. Its origins are in the Middle Ages, when the Crown assumed responsibility for managing the estates of the mentally ill and mentally handicapped. The head of the Court of Protection is called the Master. People whose affairs are managed by the court are referred to in the legislation as "patients", although the term "clients" is now used in some documentation.

The court shares premises with the Public Guardianship Office (PGO) which in April 2001 replaced the Public Trust Office. The PGO provides administrative support for the court. It is responsible for the overall running of patients' financial affairs in conjunction with receivers, and for the paperwork involved in the registration of enduring powers of attorney (see section 4.1.5). The PGO looks after the affairs of around 25 000 patients. Its average annual intake of new receivership cases is about 5000, together with a further 1000 cases where "Short Orders" are made directing the management of patients' financial affairs without appointing a receiver. The number of applications for registration of enduring powers of attorney is around 15 000 per year.[19]

It is government policy to make the Court of Protection more accessible to the public by providing it with a regional presence. Since 1 October 2001, a district judge sitting as a part-time Deputy Master of the Court of Protection has heard contentious matters at Preston Combined Court. Further appointments of Deputy Masters to hear cases in other parts of England and Wales are likely to follow.

The Court of Protection deals with the appointment of receivers and decides any contentious issues and the more serious questions arising in receivership cases. If it requires a specialist opinion about a person's mental capacity, the court may instruct one of the Lord Chancellor's Visitors to visit the patient and produce a report. There are six medical visitors. Each is a senior consultant psychiatrist, and each is responsible for a particular area of England and Wales. The main function of a receiver appointed by the Court of Protection is to receive and deal with the patient's income. If, however, the order appointing the receiver so permits, he or she has the authority to do anything necessary to ensure the proper management of the patient's property and affairs.

If an order has been made without a hearing, a request may be made for a hearing before the Master. Anyone who is aggrieved by the decision or order of the Court of Protection may appeal to a nominated High Court judge (all judges of the Chancery Division and the Family Division have been nominated). Appeals from the judge are heard by the Court of Appeal and appeals from the Court of Appeal are heard by the House of Lords.

4.2.2 Mental disorder

For a person to come within the jurisdiction of the Court of Protection it is necessary to prove two things:

- that the person is suffering from mental disorder
- that, because of the mental disorder, the person is incapable of managing and administering his or her property and affairs.[20]

These two conditions do not automatically coincide. People suffering from mental disorder might be quite capable of looking after their financial affairs and those who are not mentally disordered may be hopeless at running their affairs – they could be disorganised, uninterested, foolish, prodigal, or just lazy. To become a patient of the Court of Protection, a person's inability to manage his or her affairs must be as a result of mental disorder.

Mental disorder is defined in section 1(2) of the Mental Health Act 1983 as:

mental illness, arrested or incomplete development of mind [more commonly referred to as mental handicap or learning disability], psychopathic disorder [a persistent disorder or disability of mind which results in abnormally aggressive or seriously irresponsible conduct] and any other disorder or disability of mind [which covers disorders arising from, say, a brain injury].

Section 1(3) of the Act states that people must not be regarded as suffering from mental disorder by reason only of (a) promiscuity or other immoral conduct, (b) sexual deviancy or dependence on alcohol or drugs.

In June 2002, the government published for consultation a Mental Health Bill which, if implemented, would introduce a new definition of mental disorder. The draft Bill defines mental disorder as "any disability or disorder of mind or brain which results in an impairment or disturbance of mental functioning".[21]

Although the draft Mental Health Bill contains no proposals for the reform of Part VII of the 1983 Act concerning the Court of Protection (see section 4.2), it is proposed that this new broader definition of mental disorder will also apply to the definition of patient in Part VII once new mental health legislation is implemented.

4.2.3 Property and affairs

Assessing a patient's capacity to manage and administer his or her property and affairs is extremely subjective to the patient and the particular circumstances. The patient's ability to cope depends largely on the value and complexity of the property and affairs and the extent to which the patient may be vulnerable to exploitation. It has been held that property and affairs "means business matters, legal transactions, and other dealings of a similar kind".[22] It does not include personal matters such as where to live or decisions about medical treatment.

4.2.4 Meaning of capacity to manage property and affairs

Until 2002 there had been no reported decisions on the meaning of the term "capacity to manage property and affairs". It was generally accepted that the extent, importance and complexity of the individual's property and affairs must be taken into account.[23] Another consideration is the extent to which the person may rely upon the advice or support of others. One unreported case concerned a claim for damages in a personal injury action on behalf of a young woman who (several years earlier) had sustained a head injury in a car crash. The test of capacity to manage property and affairs was explained as follows:

> The expression "incapable of managing her own affairs and property" must be construed in a common sense way as a whole. It does not call for proof of complete incapacity ... Few people have the capacity to manage all their affairs unaided. In matters of law, particularly litigation, medicine and given sufficient resources, finance, professional advice is almost universally needed and sought ... It may be that she would have chosen, and would choose now, not to take advice, but that is not the question. The question is: is she capable of doing so? To have that capacity she requires first the insight and understanding of the fact that she has a problem in respect of which she needs advice ... Secondly, having identified the problem, it will be necessary for her to seek an appropriate adviser and to instruct him with sufficient clarity to enable him to understand the problem and to advise her appropriately ... Finally, she needs sufficient mental capacity to understand and to make decisions based upon, or otherwise give effect to such advice as she may receive.[24]

The first reported judgment on this issue was given in March 2002 in the case of *Martin Masterman-Lister v (1) Jewell (2) Home Counties Dairies and Martin Masterman-Lister v Brutton & Co.*[25] Martin Masterman-Lister was 17 years old in 1980 when the motorbike he was riding collided with a milk float. He sustained various orthopaedic injuries and a severe head injury but eventually recovered after treatment. He was able to live independently, albeit with support from his parents. In the personal injury litigation which followed, Martin's claim for damages against the driver of the milk float was finally settled in 1987. On Counsel's advice, Martin agreed to accept a reduced amount of damages (half of the full amount claimed) because it was argued that the speed at which he was driving amounted to contributory negligence on Martin's part. Several years later, Martin sought to re-open the case and seek further damages.

Generally, the Limitation Act 1980 prevents cases from being re-opened after a certain time has elapsed, except in specific circumstances. It was argued in this later action that the injuries Martin had suffered had caused him to be incapable of managing his property and affairs and he was therefore a "patient" as defined by Part 21 of the Civil Procedure Rules for the purposes of conducting litigation (see section 7.2.1) – even though this had not been raised during the original litigation. If Martin were found to be a patient, the time limits preventing the re-opening of the case would not apply. The original settlement would need to be set aside because it had not been approved by the court, as is required in the case of patients (see section 7.1), leaving the way open for Martin to pursue a claim for a higher award of damages. Everything therefore hinged on whether or not Martin was still – or ever had been – incapable of managing his property and affairs as a result of the head injury he sustained.

Mr Justice Wright considered a range of medical, witness and documentary evidence covering the 11-year period following the accident. He ruled that Martin may have been a patient for the first 3 years after the accident, but by 1983 he had recovered to the extent that he was capable of managing his own affairs and since then had not been a patient. Martin therefore had capacity at the time the settlement was agreed, so it could not be set aside and the case could not be re-opened.

In reaching his decision, the judge reviewed all of the existing authorities and guidance relating to capacity to manage property and affairs. He based his decision on the following principles.

- Legal capacity depends on understanding rather than wisdom – the quality of the decision is irrelevant so long as the person understands what he or she is deciding.
- Capacity to manage property and affairs is a question of functional capacity and essentially a subjective matter – the nature and extent of the individual's property and affairs are therefore relevant.
- Personal information must also be considered, including the condition in which the person lives, family background, family and social responsibilities and the degree of backup and support available.

This decision was upheld by the Court of Appeal,[26] which confirmed the "issue-specific nature" of the test of capacity, which must be considered in relation to the particular transaction (including its nature and complexity) under consideration. A distinction was drawn between capacity to manage day-to-day affairs, capacity to deal with the complexities of personal injury litigation, and capacity to manage a large award of damages. By way of example, Lord Justice Kennedy confirmed that in relation to an application to the Court of Protection:

> the judge must consider the totality of the property and affairs of the alleged patient and no doubt if it is shown that he lacks capacity to manage a significant part of his affairs, the court will be prepared to act, exercising control in such a way that the patient continues to have control in relation to the matters which he can handle.[27]

At the time of writing, it was understood that this case may be appealed to the House of Lords.

In personal injury actions, however, it is necessary to focus first on the person's ability to participate in the litigation rather than the whole of his or her affairs (see Chapter 7) and then to consider separately the person's capacity to manage any award of damages.

> It is not difficult to envisage claimants ... with capacity to deal with all matters and take all "lay client" decisions related to their actions up to and including a decision whether or not to settle, but lacking capacity to decide (even with advice) how to administer a large award.[28]

4.2.5 Checklist

In the High Court decision in *Masterman-Lister*, Mr Justice Wright endorsed the following checklist which was published in the first edition of this book.[29] The checklist is not intended to be exhaustive or authoritative, but gives some indication of the wide range of information which may be needed in order to make a proper assessment of a person's capacity to manage his or her property and affairs. It is worth emphasising again that the presence of a mental disorder is a pre-requisite to a conclusion that a person falls within the definition of a "patient" who lacks capacity to manage and administer his or her property and affairs.

The extent of the person's property and affairs

The extent of the person's property and affairs would include an examination of:

- a person's income and capital (including savings and the value of the home), expenditure, and liabilities
- financial needs and responsibilities
- whether there are likely to be any changes in the person's financial circumstances in the foreseeable future
- the skill, specialised knowledge, and time it takes to manage the affairs properly and whether the mental disorder is affecting the management of the assets
- whether the person would be likely to seek, understand and act on appropriate advice where needed in view of the complexity of the affairs.

Personal information

Personal information about the patient might include: age; life expectancy; psychiatric history; prospects of recovery or deterioration; the extent to which the incapacity could fluctuate; the condition in which the person lives; family background; family and social responsibilities; any cultural, ethnic or religious considerations; the degree of backup and support the person receives or could expect to receive from others.

A person's vulnerability

Other issues should be considered with the following questions.

- Could inability to manage the property and affairs lead to the person making rash or irresponsible decisions?
- Could inability to manage lead to exploitation by others – perhaps even members of the person's family?
- Could inability to manage lead to the position of other people being compromised or jeopardised?

In *Masterman-Lister* Mr Justice Wright held that "while [the above questions] are plainly proper and appropriate questions to ask, they have to be answered, in my view, in the light of the other guidance set out in the checklist".[30]

4.2.6 Proposals for law reform affecting the Court of Protection

If enacted, proposals in the Mental Incapacity Bill, which originated with recommendations from the Law Commission would significantly alter the jurisdiction of the Court of Protection. The new Court of Protection would have powers to make decisions about the personal welfare and medical treatment, as well as the property and affairs of a person without capacity.

4.3 Capacity to claim and receive social security benefits

There is a statutory mechanism through which social security benefits may be claimed on behalf of people lacking capacity to manage their own affairs. This procedure, called appointeeship, is normally used when an incapacitated person has limited assets and income only from benefits or pensions, and there is no need for more formal procedures.

4.3.1 Appointeeship

If a person is entitled to social security benefits, but is considered to be incapable of claiming and managing them, the Secretary of State for Work and Pensions can appoint an individual aged 18 or over (known as an appointee) to:

- exercise any rights and duties the claimant has under the Social Security Acts and Regulations. For example: claiming benefits; establishing "good cause" for any delay in making a claim; informing the relevant benefit office of any change in the claimant's circumstances; and appealing against the decision of an adjudication officer
- receive any benefits payable to the claimant
- deal with the money received on the claimant's behalf in the interests of the claimant and his or her dependants.

Appointeeship is governed by Regulation 33 of the Social Security (Claims and Payments) Regulations 1987 which says that an appointee may be appointed by the Secretary of State where:

- a person is, or is alleged to be, entitled to benefit, whether or not a claim for benefit has been made by him or on his behalf
- that person is unable for the time being to act
- no receiver has been appointed by the Court of Protection with power to claim or, as the case may be, receive benefit on his behalf.[31]

The test of capacity is therefore that the person is "for the time being unable to act". The Regulation does not define this phrase, but internal guidance published by the Department for Work and Pensions (DWP) suggests that people may be unable to act "for example, because of senility or mental illness".[32]

Some decisions of the Social Security Commissioners have considered the claimant's capacity, mainly in relation to the level of the claimant's understanding when making a claim which resulted in overpayment,[33] but there are no formal legal criteria which specify the capacity required. It has been suggested that in order to have the capacity to claim, receive and deal with benefits, an individual should be able to:

- understand the basis of possible entitlement (presumably with advice where necessary)
- understand and complete the claim form
- respond to correspondence relating to social security benefits
- collect or receive the benefits
- manage the benefits in the sense of knowing what the money is for
- choose whether to use it for that purpose and if so, how.[34]

The application for the appointment of an appointee,[35] which is usually completed by the person applying to be appointed, states "You may be asked to produce medical evidence of the claimant's inability to manage his own affairs". There is no standard form of medical certificate, however, and in the majority of cases, medical evidence is not required.

The Secretary of State can revoke an appointment at any time, and there is no right of appeal to a tribunal against the Secretary of State's refusal to appoint a particular individual as appointee or against the revocation of such an appointment. Appointees have no authority to deal with the claimant's capital. If the claimant has capital and it needs to be applied or invested, an application should be made to the Public Guardianship Office for directions as to how to proceed.

4.4 Protection from financial abuse

People who are, or are becoming, incapable of dealing with their own financial affairs are particularly vulnerable to abuse, which can range from outright fraud to inadvertent mishandling of money by attorneys or appointees who are not fully aware of what they can or cannot do. Professional advisers have an important role to play in protecting incapacitated people from the risk of abuse, particularly at the time of assessing capacity.

When carrying out an assessment of capacity to manage property and affairs, the following checklist may be helpful to professional advisers in assessing risk and guarding against possible abuse.

- Never express an opinion on a person's capacity without first seeing him or her for that purpose.
- Make sure the correct test of capacity is applied in relation to the particular transaction being considered, taking account of the individual circumstances, and in particular, the vulnerability of the person being assessed.
- Be careful of mistaking the person's ability to express a choice (such as who should be the attorney) for the ability to understand the nature and effect of a particular transaction (such as making an enduring power of attorney).
- In assessing the ability to understand, make sure the person is aware of and able to appreciate not only the benefits, but also the risks involved in the particular transaction.
- Always give reasons for deciding why a person has or does not have the required degree of understanding.[36]

References and notes

1   Powers of Attorney Act 1971 s10(1). Enduring Powers of Attorney Act 1985, s3(2).
2   Enduring Powers of Attorney (Prescribed Form) Regulations 1990.
3   Enduring Powers of Attorney Act 1985, s4.
4   Ibid: Schedule 1. Paragraph 2(1).
5   Re K, Re F [1988] 1 All ER 358.
6   Ibid: 363d–f.
7   In 2000, the period between creation of an EPA and application to register was less than 1 month in 7% of cases and 1–3 months in 11%. Quoted in Lush D. *Cretney and Lush on enduring powers of attorney, 5th ed*. Bristol: Jordans, 2001:9.
8   Re Beaney (deceased) [1978] All ER 595.
9   Re W (Enduring Power of Attorney) [2001] 1 FLR 832: paragraphs 23 and 25.
10 Kenward v Adams (1975) The Times, 29 November 1975.
11 The Law Society Mental Health & Disability Committee. *Enduring powers of attorney: guidelines for solicitors*. London: The Law Society, 1999.
12 Enduring Powers of Attorney Act 1985, s6(5).
13 Re W (Enduring Power of Attorney) [2001]. Op cit.
14 Rees D. Enduring powers of attorney. In: Lush D, ed. *Heyward and Massey: Court of Protection practice, 13th ed*. London: Sweet and Maxwell, 2002: paragraph 6–042.
15 Law Commission. *Mental incapacity*. London: HMSO, 1995: Part VII (Law Com No 231).
16 Lord Chancellor's Department. *Who decides? Making decisions on behalf of mentally incapacitated adults*. London: HMSO, 1997 (Cm 3803).
17 Lord Chancellor's Department. *Making decisions: the government's proposals for making decisions on behalf of mentally incapacitated adults*. London: The Stationery Office, 1999 (Cm 4465).
18 Court of Protection Rules 2001, rule 2(1).
19 Masterman-Lister v Brutton & Co and Jewell & Home Counties Dairies [2003] 3 All ER 162: 169.
20 Mental Health Act 1983, s94(2).
21 Department of Health. *Draft Mental Health Bill*. London: The Stationery Office, 2002: Clause 2(6) (Cm 5538–I).
22 F v West Berkshire Health Authority [1989] 2 All ER 545: 554d.
23 Re CAF (1962) (unreported) quoted in: Martin Masterman-Lister v (1) Jewell (2) Home Counties Dairies and Martin Masterman-Lister v Brutton & Co [2002] Lloyds Rep Med 239:244.
24 White v Fell (1987) (unreported) quoted in: Martin Masterman-Lister v (1) Jewell (2) Home Counties Dairies and Martin Masterman-Lister v Brutton & Co [2002]. Op cit:245.
25 Martin Masterman-Lister v (1) Jewell (2) Home Counties Dairies and Martin Masterman-Lister v Brutton & Co [2002]. Op cit.
26 Masterman-Lister v Brutton & Co and Jewell & Home Counties Dairies [2003]. Op cit.
27 Ibid: 171.
28 Ibid: 173.
29 Martin Masterman-Lister v (1) Jewell (2) Home Counties Dairies and Martin Masterman-Lister v Brutton & Co [2002] Lloyds Rep Med 239: 245.
30 Ibid: 246.
31 Social Security (Claims and Payments) Regulations 1987: SI 1987 No 1968.

32 Department for Work and Pensions. *Decision makers guide*. London: DWP (updated regularly): paragraph 02308. (Available on line at http://www.dwp.gov.uk)

33 See, for example, the following reported decisions of the Social Security Commissioners: R(A) 1/95; R(IS) 14/96; R(IS) 5/00 (available on line at http://www.osscsc.gov.uk).

34 Lavery R, Lundy L. The social security appointee system. *J Social Welf Law* 1994;**16**:313–27:316.

35 Department for Work and Pensions. *Application for appointment to act on behalf of someone else*. Form BF56.

36 This checklist has been adapted from Lush D. Managing the financial affairs of mentally incapacitated persons in the United Kingdom and Ireland. In: Jacoby R, Oppenheimer C, eds. *Psychiatry in the elderly, 3rd ed.* Oxford: Oxford University Press, 2002.

5 Capacity to make a will

5.1 Introduction

A will is a document in which the maker (called the "testator" if he is a man, and the "testatrix" if she is a woman) appoints an executor to deal with his or her affairs when the person dies, and describes how the person's estate is to be distributed after death. The maker of a will must be aged 18 or over. A will comes into operation only on the maker's death. Until then the person can revoke the will or make a new one at any time, provided that he or she still has the capacity to do so. The making of a new will normally revokes any previous will, provided the person making the will had the capacity to do so (see section 5.6 on capacity to revoke a will).

Someone who dies without leaving a valid will is said to die intestate. The person responsible for sorting out an intestate's affairs is called an administrator, and that person has a duty to distribute the estate to the intestate's relatives in the shares set out in the Administration of Estates Act 1925 (as amended).

About 10% of the wills made in England and Wales are home-made – handwritten or typed by the person making it – usually on a pre-printed form bought at a stationers or Post Office. In most cases, however, people ask a solicitor to prepare a will for them. Solicitors instructed to prepare a will must first be satisfied that the client has the required capacity (see section 5.2), assisted by a medical opinion where necessary (see section 5.4). The solicitor discusses the client's circumstances; advises him or her of the various options; prepares a draft will based on these discussions; and sends a copy of the draft to the client for approval. The draft is then approved or amended, and the will prepared in readiness for executing (signing) in the presence of a witness.

The degree of understanding which the law requires a person making a will to have is commonly known as "testamentary capacity". People making a will should have testamentary capacity both when they give instructions to a solicitor for the preparation of the will (or, in the case of a home-made will, when they write or type it), and when they execute, or sign, the will.

5.2 Testamentary capacity

The most important case on testamentary capacity is *Banks v Goodfellow*.[1] In this case the testator, John Banks, was a bachelor in his 50s who lived with his teenaged niece, Margaret Goodfellow. He was a paranoid schizophrenic and was convinced that a grocer (who was, in fact, dead) was pursuing and persecuting him. In 1863, with his solicitor's assistance, he made a short and simple will leaving his entire estate (15 houses) to Margaret. He died in 1865 and Margaret inherited the estate.

Nobody would have questioned the validity of this will were it not for the fact that Margaret died shortly after coming into her inheritance. She was under-age and unmarried, and the 15 properties passed to her half-brother, who was not related to John Banks. The will was contested by various members of the Banks family on the grounds that, when he made the will, John had lacked testamentary capacity because of his paranoid delusions. The court held that partial unsoundness of mind, which has no influence on the way in which a testator disposes of his property, is not sufficient to make a person incapable of validly disposing of his property by will. So John Banks' will was valid.

The Lord Chief Justice set out the following criteria for testamentary capacity:

> It is essential ... that a testator shall understand the nature of the act and its effects; shall understand the extent of the property of which he is disposing; shall be able to comprehend and appreciate the claims to which he ought to give effect; and, with a view to the latter object, that no disorder of mind shall poison his affections, pervert his sense of right, or prevent the exercise of his natural faculties – that no insane delusion shall influence his will in disposing of his property and bring about a disposal of it which, if the mind had been sound, would not have been made.[2]

The first three elements (understanding the nature of the act, its effects, and the extent of the property being disposed of) involve the will-maker's understanding: in other words, the ability to receive and evaluate information which may possibly be communicated by others. The final test (being able to comprehend the claims to which he or she ought to give effect) goes beyond understanding and requires the person making the will to be able to distinguish and compare potential beneficiaries and arrive at some form of judgment. A person making a will can, if mentally capable, ignore the claims of relatives and other potential beneficiaries.

Everyone has the right to be capricious, foolish, biased or prejudiced, and it is important to remember that when someone's capacity is being assessed it is the ability to make a decision (not necessarily a sensible or wise decision) that is under scrutiny. In the case of *Bird v Luckie* the judge specifically remarked that although the law requires a person to be capable of understanding the nature and effect of an action, it does not insist that the person behaves "in such a manner as to deserve approbation from the prudent, the wise, or the good".[3]

It is not clear how far a solicitor or doctor can assist in enhancing the capacity of someone who is making a will. An explanation in broad terms and simple language of relevant basic information about the nature and effect of the will is probably in order. Within reason, it may also be appropriate to remind the person making the will of the extent of his or her assets. But the final test, being able to comprehend and appreciate the claims to which he or she ought to give effect, is one that the person must pass unaided. There is a substantial body of judicial authority which insists that "unquestionably, there must be a complete and absolute proof that the party who had so formed the will did it without any assistance"[4] and that "a disposing mind and memory is one able to comprehend, of its own initiative and volition, the essential elements of willmaking ... merely to be able to make rational responses is not enough, nor to repeat a tutored formula of simple terms".[5]

5.3 Supervening incapacity

Occasionally a person becomes ill, or his or her condition deteriorates, between giving instructions for the preparation of a will and executing it. In these circumstances, if the will has been prepared strictly in accordance with the instructions given, it may still be valid even though, when it is executed, the person merely recalls giving instructions to the solicitor and believes that the will being executed complies with those instructions. This is known as the rule in *Parker v Felgate*.[6] This case concerned a 28-year-old widow, Mrs Compton, who suffered from glomerulonephritis, or Bright's disease. In July 1882 she consulted her solicitor about making a new will. She wanted to leave £500 to her father, £250 to her brother, and the rest of her estate (about £2500) to Great Ormond Street Hospital. During August she experienced extreme renal failure. The will was drawn up on the basis of the earlier instructions, and it was signed by someone else in her presence and at her direction, as the law permits. Four days later Mrs Compton died. Her father and brother, who would have benefited on her intestacy, contested the will on the grounds that she lacked testamentary capacity when the will was executed.

The judge held that in a case of this nature three questions must be asked.

- When the will was executed, did she remember and understand the instructions she had given to her solicitor?
- If it had been thought advisable to stimulate her, could she have understood each clause of the will when it was explained to her?
- Was she capable of understanding, and did she understand, that she was executing a will for which she had previously given instructions to her solicitor?

These questions should be asked in the order of priority listed above, and if the answer to any one of them is "yes" the will shall be valid. On the evidence in this particular case the jury answered "no" to the first two questions, and "yes" to the third, and accordingly Mrs Compton's will was valid and Great Ormond Street Hospital got its legacy.

The same principle applies when the person making a will has written or typed it and that person's condition deteriorates between preparing the will and executing it.[7]

5.4 The need for medical evidence – the "golden rule"

There is a "golden rule" that a solicitor, when drawing up a will for an elderly person or someone who is seriously ill, should ensure that the will is witnessed or approved by a medical practitioner.[8] When a medical practitioner witnesses a will, there is a strong inference that the doctor has made a formal assessment of the person and reached the conclusion that he or she has the requisite capacity to make a will (see section 3.5.1). The medical practitioner should record his or her examination and findings and, where there is an earlier will, it should be examined and any proposed alterations should be discussed with the person. Doctors should not, however, be involved in an assessment of capacity to make a will, or act as witness to a will, in which they are named as a beneficiary.

Where medical opinion is sought on an assessment as to testamentary capacity, this is best achieved by careful instructions to the doctor. There is a sample letter of instruction, setting out the relevant issues, in Appendix G.

5.5 Checklist

The following checklist covers what is meant by "understanding the nature of the act and its effects", "understanding the extent of the property being disposed of" and being "able to comprehend and appreciate the claims to which a person making a will ought to give effect". It is not intended to be either authoritative or exhaustive, but gives an indication of the issues which the will-maker must be able to understand, depending on his or her individual circumstances. For the first three elements, considered below, the test of capacity involves the person's ability to receive and evaluate information which may be communicated by others, such as a solicitor. The final element of the test requires the person to exercise choice.

5.5.1 The nature of the act of making a will

People making a will should understand that:

- they will die
- the will shall come into operation on their death, but not before
- they can change or revoke the will at any time before their death, provided they have the capacity to do so.

5.5.2 The effects of making a will

People making a will should understand (and where necessary make choices in regard to):

- who should be appointed as executor(s) (and perhaps why they should be appointed)
- who gets what under the will
- whether a beneficiary's gift is outright or conditional (for example, where the beneficiary is only entitled to the income from a lump sum during his or her lifetime, or is allowed to occupy residential property for the rest of the beneficiary's life)
- that if they spend their money or give away or sell their property during their lifetime, the beneficiaries might lose out
- that a beneficiary might die before them
- whether they have already made a will and, if so, how and why the new will differs from the old one.

5.5.3 The extent of the property

It is important to note that the judge in *Banks v Goodfellow*[9] used the word extent, rather than value. Practical difficulties can arise when the investments of the person making the will are managed by somebody else and there are no recent statements or valuations. In these cases solicitors should apply a reasonableness test to any estimate the person making the will gives about the extent of his or her wealth.

People making a will should understand:

- the extent of all the property owned solely by them
- the fact that certain types of jointly owned property might automatically pass to the other joint owner, regardless of anything that is said in the will

- whether there are benefits payable on their death which might be unaffected by the terms of their will (insurance policies, pension rights, etc)
- that the extent of their property could change during their lifetime.

5.5.4 The claims of others

People making a will should be able to comprehend and appreciate the claims to which they ought to give effect. While they have the right to ignore these claims, even to the extent of being prejudiced or capricious, they must be able to give reasons for preferring some beneficiaries and, perhaps, excluding others. For example possible beneficiaries:

- may already have received adequate provision from the person
- may be financially better off than others
- may have been more attentive or caring than others
- may be in greater need of assistance because of their age, or physical or mental disabilities.

5.6 Capacity to revoke a will

When a will is revoked it is cancelled, and will no longer come into effect on its maker's death. A will can be revoked in three ways.

- If the person who made it subsequently gets married, the will is automatically revoked by operation of law, unless it was specifically made in contemplation of that marriage (capacity to consent to marriage is discussed in section 10.4). If a person who lacks testamentary capacity marries (thereby revoking a previous will) it may be necessary to apply to the Court of Protection for the making of a statutory will (see section 5.7).
- Making a will or signing a document which expressly states that the earlier will is revoked. In this case the usual rules on testamentary capacity apply.
- With the intention of revoking the will, the maker personally burns, tears or destroys it, or authorises

somebody else to burn, tear or destroy it in the maker's presence.

The capacity required to revoke a will by destroying it was considered in the case of *Re Sabatini*.[10] In June 1940 Mrs Ruth Sabatini executed a will in which she left a few legacies to various friends and relatives, and the rest of her estate to her favourite nephew, Anthony. On 16 September 1965 she tore up this will. On 24 November 1965 she was diagnosed as suffering from Alzheimer's disease. She died in May 1966, aged 91. If the will had been validly revoked, Mrs Sabatini would have died intestate, and the whole of her estate (worth just over £50 000) would have been distributed among eight nephews and nieces, each getting an equal share. Since the original 1940 will had been destroyed, Anthony applied for probate of a carbon copy which would give him legal authority to deal with his aunt's estate according to that will. He realised that the burden was on him to prove that his aunt was not of sound mind, memory, and understanding when she tore up her will. He produced compelling medical evidence to support his case.

The barrister representing the other seven nephews and nieces put forward the argument that a lower standard of capacity, a lesser degree of concentration, was acceptable when a will is destroyed, and that a person who was incapable of making a new will might understand that a beneficiary had become unworthy of his or her inheritance and wish to deprive the beneficiary of it by tearing up the will and dying intestate. The judge rejected this argument, and said that as a general rule an individual must have the same standard of mind and memory and the same degree of understanding when destroying a will as when making one. Taking all the evidence in this case, and regarding the events of 16 September in the light of what had happened before and Mrs Sabatini's condition afterwards, the only possible conclusion was that the destruction of her will was not "a rational act rationally done". She did not have the capacity to revoke her will, and the carbon copy of the 1940 will was accepted for the purpose of granting probate.

The Sabatini case establishes that a person who intends to revoke his or her will must be capable of:

- understanding the nature of the act of revoking a will
- understanding the effect of revoking the will (this might even involve a greater understanding of the operation of the intestacy rules than is necessary for the purpose of making a will, although there is no direct authority on the point and it would be extremely difficult to prove retrospectively)
- understanding the extent of his or her property
- comprehending and appreciating the claims to which he or she ought to give effect.

5.7 Statutory wills

If a person is both (a) incapable, by reason of mental disorder, of managing and administering his or her property and affairs, and (b) incapable of making a valid will for himself or herself, an application can be made to the Court of Protection for what is known as a statutory will to be drawn up and executed on the person's behalf.[11] The court requires medical evidence of both types of incapacity (see section 4.2). The fact that a person is a patient of the Court of Protection does not mean that the person lacks testamentary capacity. If the person has testamentary capacity a solicitor can be instructed and the will drawn up under the direction of the Court of Protection.

In the case *Re D(J)* it was held that, when deciding what provisions should be included in a statutory will, the Court of Protection "must seek to make the will which the actual patient, acting reasonably, would have made if notionally restored to full mental capacity, memory and foresight". The judge laid down the following five principles which the court must have regard to:

(i) it is to be assumed that the patient is having a brief lucid interval at the time when the will is made; (ii) it is to be assumed that during the lucid interval the patient has a full knowledge of the past and a full realisation that, as soon as the will is executed, he or she will relapse into the actual mental state that previously existed, with the prognosis as it actually is; (iii) it is the actual patient who has to be considered and not a hypothetical patient; (iv) during the hypothetical lucid interval the patient is to be envisaged as being advised by competent solicitors; and (v) in all normal cases the patient is to be envisaged as taking a broad brush to the claims on his or her bounty, rather than an accountant's pen.[12]

The court must also consider the benefit of the patient's family and make provision for other persons or purposes (for example, donations to charities) for whom or for which the person might provide if not mentally disordered.[13]

References and notes

1   Banks v Goodfellow (1870) LR 5 QB 549.
2   Ibid: 565.
3   Bird v Luckie (1850) 8 Hare 301.
4   Cartwright v Cartwright (1793) 1 Phill Ecc 90: 101.
5   Leger v Poirier [1944] 3 DLR 1: 11–12.
6   Parker v Felgate (1883) 8 PD 171.
7   In the Estate of Wallace: Solicitor of the Duchy of Cornwall v Batten [1952] TLR 925.
8   See: Kenward v Adams (1975) The Times, 29 November 1975. Buckenham v Dickinson [1997] CLY 661.
9   Banks v Goodfellow (1870). Op cit.
10 Re Sabatini (1970) 114 SJ 35.
11 Mental Health Act 1983, s96 (1)(e).
12 Re D(J) [1982] 2 All ER 37: 42–43.
13 Re C (A Patient) [1991] 3 All ER 866.

6 Capacity to make a gift

6.1 Introduction

It is not uncommon for people (especially older people) to give away some or most of their assets to others – usually to their children or grandchildren. Often a gift is made to reduce the amount of tax payable on their death, and the law regards tax avoidance – as distinct from tax evasion – as an entirely legitimate exercise. Sometimes a gift is made for other reasons: perhaps to prevent assets falling into the hands of creditors on bankruptcy, or to enable the giver to claim social security benefits or to be funded by a local authority if the person has to go into a residential care home or nursing home. Parliament has anticipated most of these schemes and the relevant legislation usually contains lengthy anti-avoidance provisions which could render such gifts ineffective. The Law Society issues guidance for solicitors on the factors to be taken into account when advising clients about making gifts of property, in particular the implications for future liability to pay for long-term care.[1]

Anyone who is asked to assess whether a person is capable of making a gift should (a) not let the underlying purpose or motive affect the assessment, unless it is so perverse as to cast doubt on capacity, and (b) be satisfied that the giver is acting freely and voluntarily, and that no-one is pressurising the person into making a gift. A professional who is the likely recipient should not be involved in an assessment of capacity to make a gift.

6.2 The test of capacity

The most important case on capacity to make a gift is *Re Beaney (Deceased).*[2] In that case a 64-year-old widow with three grown up children owned and lived in a three-bedroomed semi-detached house. Her elder daughter lived with her. In May 1973, a few days after being admitted to hospital suffering from advanced dementia, the widow signed a deed of gift transferring the house to her elder daughter. The widow died intestate the following year. Her son and younger daughter applied successfully to the court for a declaration that the transfer of the house was void and of no effect because their mother was mentally incapable of making such a gift. The judge in the case set out the following criteria for capacity to make a lifetime gift:

> The degree or extent of understanding required in respect of any instrument is relative to the particular transaction which it is to effect ... Thus, at one extreme, if the subject-matter and value of a gift are trivial in relation to the donor's other assets, a low degree of understanding will suffice. But, at the other, if its effect is to dispose of the donor's only asset of value and thus, for practical purposes, to pre-empt the devolution of his estate under [the donor's] will or ... intestacy, then the degree of understanding required is as high as that required for a will, and the donor must understand the claims of all potential donees and the extent of the property to be disposed of.

It is arguable that, when someone makes a substantial gift, a further point should be considered: namely, the effect that disposing of the asset could have on the donor for the rest of his or her life.

6.3 Checklist

This checklist includes some of the points that may need to be considered in order to establish whether someone has the capacity to make a lifetime gift of a substantial asset. Some elements may involve assessing the person's ability to receive and evaluate information which may possibly be communicated by others, such as a solicitor or other adviser. Others involve the person's ability to exercise personal choice. A lower level of capacity is sufficient where the gift is insignificant in the context of the person's assets as a whole.

6.3.1 The nature of the transaction

People making a gift should understand the following about the nature of the transaction:

- that it is a gift (rather than, say, a loan or a mortgage advance or the acquisition of a stake or share in the recipient's business or property)
- whether they expect to receive anything in return

- whether they intend the gift to take effect immediately or at some later date – perhaps on death
- who the recipient is
- whether they have already made substantial gifts to the recipient or others
- whether the gift is a one-off, or part of a larger transaction or series of transactions
- the fact that if the gift is outright they will not be able to ask for the asset to be returned
- the underlying purpose of the transaction.

6.3.2 The effect of the transaction

People who make a gift should understand the possible effects of the transaction, such as:

- the effect that making the gift will have on their own standard of living in the future, having regard to all the circumstances including their age, life expectancy, income, financial resources, financial responsibilities and financial needs
- the effect that receiving the gift may have on the recipient.

6.3.3 The extent of the property

People who make a gift should understand the following about the extent of the property:

- that the subject matter of the gift belongs to them, and that they are entitled to dispose of it
- the extent (and possibly the value) of the property comprised in the gift in relation to all the circumstances and, in particular, in the context of their other assets.

6.3.4 The claims to which the giver ought to give effect

People who make a gift should be able to comprehend and appreciate the claims of the potential beneficiaries under their will or intestacy. For instance, they must appreciate:

- the effect the gift could have on other beneficiaries
- why the recipient is more deserving than others (for example, the recipient may be less well-off financially, may have devoted more time and attention to caring for the

person, or may be in need of greater assistance because of age, or physical or mental disability)

- whether it is necessary to compensate others, perhaps by making a new will
- whether there was any bias or favouritism towards the recipient before making the gift.

6.4 Gifts made by attorneys

An attorney acting on behalf of the donor of an enduring power (see section 4.1) has limited authority to make gifts provided that (a) there is nothing in the power itself which prohibits the attorney from making gifts, and (b) the value of each gift is not unreasonable, having regard to all the circumstances and – in particular – the size of the donor's estate.[3] Attorneys can only make gifts to:

- a charity to which the donor has made gifts, or might be expected to make gifts if he or she were not mentally disordered
- any person (including the attorney) who is related to or connected with the donor, provided that the gift is of a seasonal nature, or made on the occasion of a birth or marriage, or on the anniversary of a birth or marriage.

These rules apply regardless of whether the enduring power of attorney is registered or unregistered, but an attorney cannot make gifts (unless authorised to do so by the Court of Protection) while the power is in the course of being registered. If the power is registered and the attorney wishes to make more substantial gifts or gifts to people who are not related to or connected with the donor, or on an occasion other than a birth or marriage or birthday or wedding anniversary, the attorney should apply for an order of the Court of Protection (see also sections 4.2 and 6.5).

6.5 Gifts made on behalf of Court of Protection patients

A gift, or loan, or any other financial transaction in which a gift element is proposed on behalf of a patient for whom a receiver has been appointed, gifts which the patient can afford (because they come from surplus income or capital and are insignificant in the context of his or her assets as a whole) up to a ceiling of £15 000, are usually considered and allowed by the Public Guardianship Office on an application by letter only. In other words, neither attendance at court nor the making of a formal application is necessary.

If the proposed gift does not fall within the above parameters, a formal application must be made to the Court of Protection. A hearing will be arranged and the court will allow or prohibit the gift after considering all the evidence.

6.6 Risk of financial abuse

People who are (or are becoming) incapable of looking after their own affairs are at particular risk of financial abuse and one of the easiest forms of abuse is the improper gifting of their money or other assets. This may be where vulnerable people are persuaded to give away money or property without being fully aware of the circumstances, or having the capacity to do so, or when people appointed to act on their behalf (such as attorneys or appointees) abuse their position of trust (see section 4.4). The careful assessment of capacity to make a gift is therefore an important safeguard against financial abuse.

Where medical opinion is sought on an assessment of capacity to make a gift, this is best achieved by careful instructions to the doctor. Appendix G is a sample letter of instruction which can be adapted for capacity to make a gift.

References and notes

1 The Law Society Mental Health & Disability Committee. *Gifts of property: implications for future liability to pay for long-term care.* London: The Law Society, 2000.
2 Re Beaney (Deceased) [1978] 2 All ER 595: 601f–h.
3 Enduring Powers of Attorney Act, s 3(5).

7 Capacity to litigate

7.1 Introduction

People who lack mental capacity may become parties to proceedings in the High Court of Justice and the county courts, as well as in the Court of Protection (see section 4.2). If they lack the capacity to give instructions to lawyers on the conduct of the litigation (see section 2.1), a procedure is needed to enable the proceedings to continue by appointing someone else to give instructions and otherwise act on their behalf. These procedures are to be found in the relevant rules for the type of proceedings, which are:

- Civil Procedure Rules 1998 Part 21
- Family Proceedings Rules 1991 Part IX
- Insolvency Rules 1986 Part 7 Chapter 7
- Court of Protection Rules 2001 rule 14.

For people who are already patients of the Court of Protection, authorisation must first be obtained from that court for legal proceedings to be conducted in the name of the patient or on his or her behalf.[1] These provisions (which also apply to children) ensure that, where appropriate:

- incapacitated adults or children (both referred to in the context of legal proceedings as "persons under disability") are represented by a suitable adult
- compromises and settlements agreed on their behalf are approved by the court
- there is supervision of any money recovered.

Any proceedings involving a person under disability conducted without such a representative are likely to be invalid and any settlement set aside, unless the court retrospectively gives approval.

The adult litigant who lacks capacity is referred to as a "patient" (see section 7.2.1), although a wider definition of an "incapacitated person" is used in insolvency proceedings (see section 7.2.2). The representative in civil proceedings is known as a "litigation friend". In family proceedings and in the Court of Protection, the term used is "next friend" if bringing the proceedings or "guardian ad litem" if responding to them. For simplicity, in this chapter "litigation friend" should be understood to include "next friend" and "guardian ad litem".

There is no procedure for the appointment of a litigation friend in the Magistrates (Family Proceedings) Court. Where family proceedings are commenced in that court and a litigation friend is required, the case should be transferred up to the County Court.

Solicitors asked to act on behalf of a person under disability should ensure that a suitable person is put forward for appointment as litigation friend. The appointment is made by the court that will hear the proceedings. Care should be taken to select a litigation friend who has no actual or potential conflict of interest with the patient. In most cases, a relative, friend or someone with a close connection with the patient will act as litigation friend. Where a receiver has already been appointed to manage a patient's affairs (see section 4.2), the Court of Protection normally authorises the receiver to act as litigation friend. An attorney acting under a registered enduring power of attorney (see section 4.1.2) may also be a suitable person. Where there is no suitable person willing and able to act as litigation friend, the Official Solicitor to the Supreme Court will consider accepting appointment, but should first be consulted and should give consent. Further information on the role of the Official Solicitor is given in Appendix B.

7.2 The test of capacity

7.2.1 Patients

A "patient" is defined by the Civil Procedure Rules 1998 as "a person who by reason of mental disorder within the meaning of the Mental Health Act 1983 is incapable of managing and administering his own affairs".[2]

Before the Civil Procedure Rules were introduced, the relevant definition in the former Rules of the Supreme Court 1965, Order

80 (for the High Court) and County Court Rules 1981, Order 10 (for the county courts) concluded with the words: "incapable of managing and administering his property and affairs". This wording is still used in the Family Proceedings Rules 1991[3] and by the Court of Protection[4] but it is not thought that there is any difference between the two tests in practice.

There are three general categories of person who come within this definition of patient, namely those with a mental illness, those with learning disabilities, and those with brain damage. In Court of Protection proceedings, the majority are likely to be older people suffering from senile dementia which is a form of mental illness. In other types of proceedings, such as personal injury actions, it is possible for a child also to be a patient and this may be relevant if that condition will continue into adulthood (for example a child with severe learning disability or brain damage at birth).

Although mental disorder is defined under mental health legislation which primarily deals with compulsory treatment, the test of capacity to litigate relates to a person's ability to manage his or her affairs (see section 7.3.2), and not to any need for treatment for mental disorder.

7.2.2 Insolvency proceedings

A more comprehensive definition of an "incapacitated person" is available for insolvency proceedings, namely a person who is incapable of managing and administering his or her property and affairs either (a) by reason of mental disorder within the meaning of the Mental Health Act 1983; or (b) due to physical affliction or disability.[5]

The emphasis is thus on the person's incapacity, with a wider definition and different causes of incapacity accepted in insolvency proceedings compared with other types of litigation. It may be assumed, however, that the approach to assessing the person's mental incapacity (as opposed to physical disability) is the same.

7.3 Applying the test

There is a presumption of capacity so the burden of proof rests on those asserting incapacity. If there is clear evidence that the person has been incapacitated for a considerable period (for example following a road accident) then the burden of proof may be more easily discharged, but it remains on whoever asserts incapacity. The test is applied on the balance of probabilities, so it is not necessary to be satisfied beyond reasonable doubt that the person lacks capacity. See Part II for an explanation of these legal principles.

When considering whether an individual is incapable of personally conducting legal proceedings (other than insolvency proceedings) the following three-stage test should be applied.

1 Is he or she mentally disordered?
2 Is he or she incapable of managing and administering his or her own affairs?
3 Does the incapacity result from the mental disorder?

There are two distinct components, namely being mentally disordered, and being incapable of managing affairs. If one of these is present but there is doubt about the other, it may be appropriate to ask the court to decide whether the second component is satisfied as a preliminary issue in the legal proceedings. When a person is treated as a patient he is deprived of important rights and there is potential for a breach of the Human Rights Act 1998, yet there is no requirement under the various rules (listed in section 7.1) for a judicial determination of capacity. The final decision as to capacity rests with the court, however, which should ensure that the individual concerned is given an opportunity to make representations unless the lack of capacity is beyond doubt, and investigate the question of capacity whenever there is any reason to suspect that it may be absent.

When applying the test of capacity, evidence from the person concerned, whether admitting or denying incapacity, cannot be regarded as being of great weight. Expert evidence will normally be required, which could be from a doctor, psychologist, nurse or social worker, depending on the type of case and the circumstances of the person alleged to lack capacity. The judge may be assisted by seeing the individual but this may not always be appropriate. If the issue of capacity is contested, medical evidence will be required (especially with respect to the existence and effect of mental disorder).

Obtaining medical evidence can present real difficulties, especially if the person being assessed refuses to cooperate (see section 2.4). Where there are practical difficulties in obtaining medical evidence the Official Solicitor may be consulted and will try to assist (see Appendix B). A doctor who is asked to express an opinion as to whether a person is incapable of bringing or defending court proceedings should be provided with sufficient information as to the extent and nature of those proceedings, as well as the medical background.

7.3.1 Mental disorder

"Mental disorder" is defined by the Mental Health Act 1983 as "mental illness, arrested or incomplete development of mind, psychopathic disorder and any other disorder or disability of mind".[6] But nothing in the definition is to be construed as implying that a person may be dealt with as suffering from mental disorder by reason only of promiscuity or other immoral conduct, sexual deviancy, or dependence on alcohol or drugs (see section 4.2.2).

7.3.2 The meaning of "affairs"

The courts have held that "affairs" in this context is restricted to "business matters, legal transactions and other dealings of a similar kind";[7] it does not extend to personal and healthcare matters. When linked with "property" it can be seen that broadly speaking we are talking about "financial affairs". It should not be overlooked that it is the patient's own affairs that must be considered and not financial affairs in general. Although it is not specifically stated in the wording of the various rules governing legal proceedings, the Court of Appeal has held in the case of *Masterman-Lister v Brutton & Co and Jewell & Home Counties Dairies* that the test of capacity is "issue specific" and, in the context of litigation, relates to capacity to manage the particular legal proceedings rather than the whole of the person's affairs.[8] The details of that case are set out in section 4.2.4.

7.3.3 Incapacity

One of the problems when considering capacity is the extent to which the person may rely upon the advice or support of others. This was discussed in the unreported case of *White v Fell*, which considered the capacity of a person who had previously suffered head injuries. The test to be applied was explained as follows:

> The expression "incapable of managing her own affairs and property" must be construed in a common sense way as a whole. It does not call for proof of complete incapacity ... Few people have the capacity to manage all their affairs unaided. In matters of law, particularly litigation, medicine, and given sufficient resources, finance, professional advice is almost universally needed and sought ... It may be that she would have chosen, and would choose now, not to take advice, but that is not the question. The question is: is she capable of doing so?[9]

In the very similar *Masterman-Lister* case, it was subsequently held that legal capacity depends on understanding rather than wisdom; the quality of the decision is irrelevant as long as the person understands what is being decided and the likely effects of this action.[10] It is not the task of the courts to prevent those who have the mental capacity to make rational decisions from making decisions which others may regard as rash or irresponsible. The test of capacity for legal proceedings thus becomes:

> ... whether the party is capable of understanding, with the assistance of such proper explanation from legal advisers and experts in other disciplines as the case may require, the issues on which his consent or decision is likely to be necessary in the course of those proceedings.[11]

As indicated in the case of *White v Fell* mentioned above, capacity to litigate requires the person:

- to have "insight and understanding of the fact that ... [he or she] has a problem in respect of which ... [he or she] needs advice"
- to be able to instruct an appropriate adviser "with sufficient clarity to enable ... [the adviser] to understand the problem and advise ... [him or her] appropriately"
- "to understand and make decisions based upon, or otherwise give effect to, such advice as ... [he or she] may receive".[12]

The Court of Appeal confirmed this approach in *Masterman-Lister* but also stressed that the test includes the ability to weigh information (and advice) in the balance as part of the process of understanding and acting on that advice.[13]

7.4 The representative in legal proceedings

7.4.1 Suitability of representatives

In civil proceedings, the criteria whereby someone may be regarded as suitable for appointment as litigation friend (other than the Official Solicitor or person authorised by the Court of Protection) are that the person:

- can fairly and competently conduct proceedings on behalf of the patient
- has no interest adverse to that of the patient
- (where the patient is a claimant) undertakes to pay any costs which the patient may be ordered to pay in relation to the proceedings, subject to any right to be repaid from the assets of the patient.[14]

In family proceedings, a next friend or guardian ad litem (other than the Official Solicitor or a person authorised by the Court of Protection) appointed under the Family Proceedings Rules must file a solicitor's certificate that he or she has no interest in the cause or matter in question adverse to that of the person under disability and is a proper person to be next friend or guardian ad litem.[15]

7.4.2 Role of representatives

It is the duty of a litigation friend "fairly and competently to conduct proceedings on behalf of a ... patient. He must have no interest in the proceedings adverse to that of the ... patient and all steps and decisions he takes in the proceedings must be taken for the benefit of the ... patient".[16]

7.5 Implications of incapacity

A person who is treated as a patient in litigation does not automatically have to become a Court of Protection patient and this will depend on what the position may be after the proceedings are concluded (for example if damages are awarded). Similarly, the fact that the litigant is considered capable of giving instructions for the conduct of the proceedings does not automatically mean that the Court of Protection will not need to be involved if substantial damages are awarded.

Once it becomes clear that significant damages or compensation are to be awarded (for example in a personal injury claim or the distribution of assets on a divorce) then an application should be made to the Court of Protection for the appointment of a receiver if the litigant lacks capacity to manage these funds (see section 4.2.1). This avoids unnecessary delay in enabling the money to be dealt with. In many cases the litigation friend (or next friend in family proceedings) becomes the receiver, but this is not essential. Conversely (as indicated in section 7.1) if a receiver had already been appointed, he or she will normally be the representative for the purpose of bringing any proceedings.

References and notes

1 Mental Health Act 1983, s96(1)(i).
2 Civil Procedure Rules 1998, Part 21, rule 1(2)(b).
3 Family Proceedings Rules 1991, rule 9.1(1).
4 Mental Health Act 1983, s94(2).
5 Insolvency Rules 1986, rule 7.43(2).
6 Mental Health Act 1983, s1(2).
7 F v West Berkshire Health Authority [1989] 2 All ER 545: 554d.
8 Masterman-Lister v Brutton & Co and Jewell & Home Counties Dairies [2003] 3 All ER 162: 173
9 White v Fell (1987) (unreported) quoted in: Masterman-Lister v Brutton & Co and Jewell & Home Counties Dairies [2003]. Op cit: 170.
10 Martin Masterman-Lister v (1) Jewell (2) Home Counties Dairies and Martin Masterman-Lister v Brutton & Co [2002] Lloyds Rep Med 239: 244.
11 Masterman-Lister v Brutton & Co and Jewell & Home Counties Dairies [2003]. Op cit: 188.
12 White v Fell (1987). Op cit.
13 Masterman-Lister v Brutton & Co and Jewell & Home Counties Dairies [2003]. Op cit: 172.
14 Civil Procedure Rules 1998, rule 21.4(3).
15 Family Proceedings Rules 1991, rule 9.2(7).
16 Civil Procedure Rules 1998, Practice Direction 21, paragraph 2.1.

8 Capacity to enter into a contract

8.1 Introduction

It is difficult to generalise about an individual's contractual capacity. Without really being aware of it, most people enter into some sort of contract every day, such as purchasing groceries, buying a bus ticket or train ticket, or depositing clothes at the dry-cleaners. Some general rules apply to each of these contracts, as well as to more complicated written agreements with several pages of small print.

8.2 General rules

The starting point is that there is a presumption of capacity to enter into a contract, although of course this may be rebutted by evidence to the contrary. Unusual or eccentric behaviour does not give rise to a presumption of lack of capacity, although it may cause capacity to be questioned. Four general rules may then be identified:

- specificity
- understanding
- timing
- intention to create legal relations.

8.2.1 Specificity

The first rule is that contractual capacity relates to the specific contract, rather than to contracts in general. This means that a person could have capacity to buy a cinema ticket but not the capacity required to enter into a credit agreement with a mail-order firm.

8.2.2 Understanding

The second rule is that the person must be capable of understanding the nature and effects of the specific contract and of agreeing to it.[1] Obviously, the degree of understanding varies according to the kind of agreement involved. Some contracts require a relatively low degree of understanding (buying a bus ticket), whereas others demand a much higher level of understanding (a complex hire purchase agreement).

8.2.3 Timing

The third rule is that contractual capacity must be assessed at the time that the contract was to be entered into (not the day before, or even the hour before). The capacity of an individual can fluctuate over a period of time. Evidence of capacity or lack of capacity at a different time is irrelevant, and would be inadmissible in any court proceedings about the validity of the contract, although evidence of a general lack of capacity may be significant.

8.2.4 Intention to create legal relations

The fourth rule is that the parties must have intended to enter into a contract that is legally binding. In the case of social and domestic arrangements (for example, financial arrangements within the family) there is a presumption that there is no such intention. However, this presumption may be rebutted by evidence to the contrary.

8.3 Voidable contracts

In dealing with contracts made by people whose mental capacity is in doubt, the courts have had to counterbalance two important policy considerations. One is a duty to protect those who are incapable of looking after themselves, and the other is to ensure that other people are not prejudiced by the actions of persons who appear to have full capacity. So, people without capacity are bound by the terms of a contract they have entered into, even if it was unfair, unless it can be shown that the other party to the contract was aware of their mental incapacity or should have been aware of this.[2] For example, at some stage a person suffering from hypomania may go on a reckless shopping spree. If the shopkeeper has no reason to suspect that the customer is hypomanic, the customer is bound by the contract. But if the shopkeeper was or should have been aware of the customer's mental state, the contract is voidable, and therefore cannot be enforced (see section 8.6 for an exception).

8.4 Necessaries

A special rule applies to contracts for "necessaries". A person without mental capacity who agrees to pay for goods or services which are necessaries is legally obliged to pay a reasonable price for them. Necessaries are defined in the Sale of Goods Act 1979[3] as goods which are suitable to the person's condition in life (that is, to his or her place in society, rather than any mental or physical condition) and his or her actual requirements at the time of sale and delivery (for example, ordinary drink, food and clothing). Although the Sale of Goods Act applies to goods, similar common law rules are believed to apply to essential services such as the provision of accommodation and care in a nursing home.

Whether something is necessary or not is established in two stages by asking the following questions.

- Are the goods or services capable of being necessaries as a matter of law?
- If so, were the goods or services necessaries, given the particular circumstances of the incapacitated person who ordered them?

Case law has established that goods are not necessaries if the person's existing supply is sufficient. So, for instance, a person who buys a pair of shoes would probably be bound to pay for them, but if the same person purchased a dozen pairs, the contract might be voidable at the person's option.

A contract for necessaries cannot be enforced against a person who lacks mental capacity if it contains harsh or onerous terms. The requirement that only a reasonable price is to be paid is an extension of this principle because a reasonable price need not be the same as the agreed or sale price.[4]

8.5 Proposals for law reform

The Law Commission recommended a single statutory provision applying to the supply of both necessary goods and services to persons without capacity to contract for them.[5] This would be based on the existing law, but would allow someone acting on behalf of an incapacitated person to arrange for goods or services to be supplied (for example for milk to be delivered or roof repairs to be carried out) and to pay for them. These proposals were included in the Draft Mental Incapacity Bill published in 2003.

8.6 Court of Protection patients

If someone comes under the jurisdiction of the Court of Protection because it has been established on medical evidence that he or she is incapable, by reason of mental disorder, of managing and administering his or her property and affairs, that person (known as a "patient") cannot enter into any contract which is inconsistent with the court's powers (see section 4.2). For example, if a receiver has been given authority by the court to take over the handling of the patient's property and financial affairs, the patient cannot arrange to sell any property or purchase any goods independently of the receiver. Any such contract is void, even if the patient had contractual capacity when entering into it and the other party was unaware of the court's involvement in the patient's affairs, and even if the contract was for necessaries.[6] The patient's receiver could, however, carry out the contract on behalf of the patient if it was for his or her benefit, or could apply to the court for an order retrospectively approving the contract if it was beyond the receiver's powers.[7]

8.7 Checklist

Solicitors may wish to seek an opinion from a doctor about a client's contractual capacity, either before a contract is agreed, or retrospectively if the validity of a contract is being challenged. The solicitor should identify the specific contract to which the assessment of capacity relates. Different information is required according to the type and complexity of the contract, for example fewer details may be required concerning a contract to purchase double glazing than for a complex agreement to enter into a home income plan. The solicitor needs to provide such details as:

- the identity of the other party to the contract
- how much the client has to pay or is being paid
- when the payment will be made or received
- what is being given or received in exchange
- any important terms and conditions which affect the client's rights and liabilities
- the circumstances in which the contract was entered into (place and time of day)
- the method of communication between the parties
- any opportunity afforded to the client to reconsider the contract.

The doctor should then be asked whether the client is or was capable of understanding the nature and effect of that contract at the time a decision is or was required. Where it is considered that the client was not capable of understanding a contract made previously, which is now being challenged, the doctor should also be asked whether the client's lack of capacity should have been obvious to the other party when the contract was made.

References and notes

1 Boughton v Knight (1873) LR 3 PD 64.
2 Imperial Loan Company v Stone [1892] 1 QB 599.
3 Sale of Goods Act 1979, s3(3).
4 Sale of Goods Act 1979, s8(3).
5 Law Commission. *Mental incapacity*. London: HMSO, 1995: paragraphs 4.6–4.11. (Law Com No 231)
6 Re Walker [1905] 1 Ch 160. Re Marshall [1920] 1 Ch 284.
7 Mental Health Act 1983, s96(1)(h).

9 Capacity to vote

9.1 Entitlement to vote

The majority of people with mental health problems, whether caused by mental illness or learning disabilities, have the right to vote in parliamentary and local elections. Encouragement is needed to ensure that their names are entered on the electoral register, and that they are given every opportunity to exercise their right to vote. It is rare for doctors or lawyers to become involved in determining capacity to vote, but better knowledge of the legal position may serve to encourage more people to register and therefore to be able to vote. It is a widely held belief that any degree of learning disability or mental illness renders a person ineligible to vote. This is not true, but such a belief may result in learning disabled people or mentally ill people being excluded from the electoral register – which does disqualify them from voting.

The people entitled to vote as electors in parliamentary elections in any constituency, or in local government elections are defined in legislation as those:

- whose name appears on the relevant electoral register
- who are not subject to any legal incapacity to vote (apart from by virtue of their age)
- who are either Commonwealth citizens or citizens of the Republic of Ireland
- who are of voting age (aged 18 or over).[1]

The main factors which determine whether a learning disabled or mentally disordered person can vote are whether he or she is (a) subject to any legal incapacity to vote, and (b) has an address for registration purposes.

9.2 Legal incapacity to vote

Legal incapacity to vote was defined in a case in 1874 called *Stowe v Joliffe* as "some quality inherent in a person, which either at common law, or by statute, deprives him of the status of Parliamentary elector".[2] This definition still applies today. In relation to mental capacity, the common law applies, and refers back to cases decided in the 18th century. For example, in 1785 in the *Bedford County Case, Burgess' Case* it was held that the name of an "idiot" (somebody with severe learning disabilities) may not appear on the electoral register, and hence such a person cannot vote.[3] In 1791, case law clarified that a "lunatic" (somebody with a mental illness) can vote, though only during a lucid interval.[4] This view was confirmed in subsequent cases, with the result that mentally ill people should not be excluded from the electoral register.[5]

While the terms referred to above are offensive and have no modern clinical application, the common law still applies in determining whether someone has the capacity to vote. It is the degree of mental incapacity which is relevant in deciding whether a person's name can be entered on the electoral register, and whether he or she can vote.

There is no definition in either statute or case law of the capacity to vote. The common law sets the threshold of understanding quite low, requiring only a capacity to understand in "broad terms" the nature and effect of voting and an ability to make a choice between candidates.

9.3 Eligibility for registration

There are no provisions in law which control the registration as electors of people who have a learning disability or mental illness and who are living in the community (as opposed to living in a hospital). In practice, the decision as to whether a person with a mental disability is registered is made by that person's carer, by deciding whether or not to include the name of the disabled person on the annual canvass form which is sent to all households in September of each year. This form does not raise questions of mental capacity, so there is no reason why all adults resident in the household should not be included, unless it is clear that a person lacks the capacity to make any sort of choice because of profound learning disability. The final decision as to whether a person's name is included in the electoral roll rests with the Electoral Registration Officer (ERO) who must consider each case on its merits. There is no requirement to obtain a medical opinion although an ERO may decide that a medical opinion would be helpful in determining a person's capacity to vote. If an ERO considers someone is entitled to be registered as an elector, there is no discretion to omit that person's name from the register unless any legal incapacity to vote can be established.

Guidance issued by the Electoral Commission advises EROs in England to err – if at all – on the side of inclusion, rather than omission, in order to encourage people who have a degree of mental impairment to exercise their right to vote.[6] This places the onus on people who wish to object to the inclusion of a name to make their case, rather than requiring mentally disabled people who may be eligible to vote to use the appeals procedure in order to be registered.

9.3.1 Place of residence

The Representation of the People Act 2000, which came into effect in September 2001, introduced changes in electoral procedures and registration intended to make it easier for disabled people to register and to vote. Under previous electoral legislation, people were only able to register if they could establish their place of residence on a specific qualifying date, 10 October, each year. There were special rules relating to the voting rights of patients in "mental hospitals" as such hospitals could not be used as a place of residence for the purpose of electoral registration. The Representation of the People Act removes the annual qualifying date, and it introduced "rolling" electoral registration to enable people to be added to (or deleted from) the electoral register at any time of the year.[7]

Both voluntary (informal) and detained patients in mental hospitals (with the exception of those detained as a consequence of criminal activity) may continue to be registered for electoral purposes at their home address. If, however, their stay in hospital is so long that they have lost their residence, they may still register as electors by making a "declaration of local connection" providing a local contact address. This could be the address of the hospital, an address where they would be resident if they were not in hospital, or an address in the UK where they have lived at any time in the past.[8] Registration by declaration of local connection is also available to homeless people. It does not apply, however, to detained patients who have been convicted of a criminal offence or transferred to hospital from prison under Part III of the Mental Health Act 1983; these people, along with all sentenced prisoners, are disqualified from voting.[9]

The definition of mental hospital includes any establishment or unit whose main purpose is the reception and treatment of people suffering from any form of mental disorder.[10] This does not include hostels or other residential care homes where the treatment of residents is not the primary purpose. The definition also excludes psychiatric wards of district general hospitals and homes for elderly people.

It is for EROs to decide which hostels or residential care homes for old people, for mentally ill people, or those with learning disabilities, come within the definition of a "mental hospital". If necessary they can obtain advice from the Department of Health or local Primary Care Trust for NHS homes or hostels, or the National Care Standards Commission (the Commission for Healthcare Audit and Inspection from April 2004) for privately run institutions. For those hostels or homes which are not "mental hospitals", the ERO must decide which residents are entitled to be registered, if necessary with medical advice. The Electoral Commission guidance stipulates that the warden or person in charge of the home should not be asked to make a judgment as to which residents have the mental capacity to vote, as such a practice is not only objectionable in principle, but also is open to abuse.[11]

9.4 At the polling station

Any person whose name appears on the electoral register should be allowed to cast his or her vote unless, at the polling station on the day of the poll, it appears to the presiding officer that the elector may be so mentally incapacitated as to not have the common law capacity to vote. The presiding officer may put to the elector certain statutory questions permitted by the election rules.[12] The permitted questions are:

- Are you the person whose name appears on the register as … ?
- Have you already voted?

Although these questions are inappropriate for determining mental capacity, no further questions may be put. If the presiding officer considers that the questions are not answered satisfactorily, he or she can refuse to issue a ballot paper. If the questions are answered satisfactorily, the person must be allowed to vote.

Electors who are unable to read can ask the presiding officer to help them by marking their votes on the ballot paper, but they must be capable of giving directions to the presiding officer as to how they wish to vote. No-one is allowed to accompany an elector into the polling booth or give any other assistance in marking the ballot paper, but some voters with physical disabilities are entitled to assistance from a companion.[13]

9.5 Postal and proxy voting

The Representation of the People Act 2000 extends the provisions for permitting an elector to vote by post or by appointing a proxy to vote on his or her behalf.[14] These methods of voting are now available either at the time of registration for the period of the register, or before a particular election. Anyone on the electoral register can vote by post, which means that no check is made on their capacity when they cast their vote. No definition is given as to the mental capacity required to appoint a proxy, but it is presumed that the elector should have the common law capacity to vote and the ability to choose the person to be appointed. EROs are able to explain the procedures and provide the relevant application forms.

9.6 Conclusion

It is important that patients in hospital and residents in hostels and residential care homes are aware of their voting rights, and staff should assist them by providing information, declaration forms and absent voting forms. People with mental health problems living in the community will require help from their relatives, carers and sometimes their doctors to ensure they are not deprived unnecessarily of this most basic of civil rights.

References and notes

1   Representation of the People Act 1983, s1–2 (as amended by Representation of the People Act 2000, s1(1)).
2   Stowe v Joliffe [1874] LR9 CP 750.
3   Bedford County Case, Burgess' Case [1785] 2 Lud EC 381.
4   Oakhampton Case, Robin's Case [1791] 1 Fras 69.
5   For example: Bridgwater Case, Tucker's Case [1803] 1 Peek 101.
6   Electoral Commission. *Managing electoral services: a good practice guide for electoral administrators in England.* London: The Electoral Commission, 2002: Appendix XIV.
7   Representation of the People Act 1983, s4(6) (as amended by Representation of the People Act 2000, s1(2)).
8   Representation of the People Act 1983, s7 (as amended by Representation of the People Act 2000, s4).
9   Representation of the People Act 1983, s3A (as inserted by Representation of the People Act 2000, s2). See also: R (on the application of Pearson) v Secretary of State for Home Department, Hirst v Attorney General [2001] HRLR 39.
10 Representation of the People Act 1983, s7(6) (as amended by Representation of the People Act 2000, s4).
11 Electoral Commission. *Managing electoral services: a good practice guide for electoral administrators in England.* Op cit: Appendix XIV.
12 Representation of the People Act 1983, Schedule 1, Parliamentary Election Rules, Rule 35. Local Election (Principal Areas) Rules 1986, Rule 29. (SI 1986/2214)
13 Representation of the People Act 2000, s13 (amended the Parliamentary Election Rules to make it easier for disabled people to vote). See also: Representation of the People Regulations 2001, Regulation 12.
14 Representation of the People Act 2000, s12.

10 Capacity and personal relationships

10.1 Right to form relationships

Every person has fundamental rights which may not be infringed unless there are special and widely agreed grounds justifying such an infringement. Respect for individual rights in those matters which people can decide for themselves is embodied in national and international agreements. The United Nations Declaration on Human Rights of 1948, for example, articulates the rights of adults to freedom and equal treatment. The European Convention on Human Rights, now incorporated into UK law under the Human Rights Act 1998, says: "Everyone has the right to respect for his private and family life, his home and his correspondence";[1] and further: "Men and women of marriageable age have the right to marry and to found a family, according to the national laws governing the exercise of this right".[2]

A balance must be maintained, however, between respecting individual rights to family relationships, friendships, sexual relationships, marriage, and parenthood, and the duty of society (the state, parents, carers, and others) to protect vulnerable people from abuse. These two facets – respect for rights and protection from exploitation – are reflected in the civil and the criminal law, which take different approaches in relation to the capacity of vulnerable people to embark on intimate relationships. Whereas the civil law provides for the private rights of all citizens to enjoy family contact and personal or sexual relationships, the criminal law concentrates on providing an effective deterrent aimed at protecting vulnerable people from abuse, including sexual abuse. In both civil and criminal contexts, judgments about individuals' capacity to consent in personal relationships are extremely important. Overall, however, current case law is more concerned with the provisions available in the criminal law to protect vulnerable people from potentially abusive relationships than with their civil law rights to enter into voluntary relationships.

This difference in emphasis is echoed in the relevant tests of capacity to consent, applicable under civil and criminal law. Even though most professionals agree that it would be appropriate to have just one test – that is the civil law test of capacity to consent to sexual relations and apply it equally in criminal law proceedings – some members of the judiciary have taken a different view.[3] Obviously, the criminal law is intended to deter abuse by prosecuting and punishing those who seek to take advantage of vulnerable people. In criminal proceedings, therefore, the test of capacity to consent has developed in a context where the burden of proof is on the prosecution to prove, beyond reasonable doubt, that an offence has been committed. (The criminal law provisions are discussed further in Chapter 11.) In the rest of this chapter, the focus is on the civil law and on the aim of enabling all people to make their own voluntary decisions wherever possible. Set out here, therefore, are the specific legal provisions which relate to capacity to consent in the exercise of such rights.

10.2 Family relationships

For most people it is important to maintain family relationships (which of course vary in degree and intensity) at least with close relatives. In the context of family proceedings where children are minors, there is a general presumption of a right to a relationship between a parent and child, which should be protected so long as this is in the child's best interests. The welfare of the child is always the paramount consideration.[4] Where there is a disagreement between the parents, the right to a relationship can be enforced through a contact order under the provisions of the Children Act 1989.[5] Once children reach 18, however, the right to a relationship with their parents, or with other family members, extends for only so far as the people involved consent to it. There are no means, in legal proceedings or otherwise, of enforcing a relationship between adult family members who have capacity to decide they no longer wish the relationship to continue.

Nevertheless, the courts have been asked to intervene in cases where disputes have arisen between family members about contact with adult relatives who lack capacity to make their own decision, or to resolve disagreements about where such individuals should live. Questions of residence or contact are clearly important in enabling a relationship to continue. Until 1995, it was unclear whether the court had power under its inherent jurisdiction (powers which the courts exercise on behalf of the Crown, relating to the person and property of citizens unable to care for themselves) to hear cases concerning the personal welfare of mentally incapacitated adults, since all previous cases were concerned with medical treatment. The first case of this sort *Re S (Adult Patient: Jurisdiction)*[6] concerned a Norwegian artist, S, who was incapacitated as a result of a stoke. His estranged wife and son wanted him to be returned to Norway, out of the care of his partner with whom he had chosen to live in England before he became incapacitated. The court held that there was jurisdiction and granted an injunction to prevent S being taken abroad. This decision was upheld in the Court of Appeal.[7]

The court's jurisdiction to grant declarations as to the best interests of a mentally incapable person has been called upon on many subsequent occasions[8], and was comprehensively reviewed and confirmed in 2000 in the case *Re F (Adult: Court's Jurisdiction)*.[9] This case concerned T, an 18-year-old woman with a severe learning disability. She was one of eight children, all of whom had been in local authority care because of a serious lack of adequate parenting and exposure to sexual abuse. When T became 18, her mother wanted her to return to the family home. The local authority sought a declaration from the court that it would be in T's best interests to remain in local authority accommodation and for the local authority to restrict and supervise her contact with her mother. It was held that where there was a risk of possible harm to a mentally incapable adult, the court had power under the inherent jurisdiction to hear the issues involved and to grant declarations in the best interests of the incapacitated person. This case also upheld the court's role in ensuring compliance with the Human Rights Act in all aspects of decision making on behalf of incapacitated adults.

The court's jurisdiction in these types of cases has developed considerably and will no doubt continue to do so. For example, in the case of *Re S (Adult Patient) (Inherent Jurisdiction:*

Family Life) it was held that the parents of mentally incapacitated adults have powers under the doctrine of necessity (see section 12.4.1 for discussion of the doctrine of necessity in the context of medical treatment) to continue to assume day-to-day responsibility for the person's care. Moreover, they may make certain decisions, where appropriate in conjunction with professional advisers, about important matters including where the person should live. Where there are disputes about such decisions, the judge held that:

> The court has jurisdiction to grant whatever relief in declaratory form is necessary to safeguard and promote the incapable adult's welfare and interests. ... the court has, and in my judgment always has had, power to declare that some specified person is to be, in relation to specified matters, what is, in effect, a surrogate decision-maker for the incapable adult.[10]

At the time of writing it is understood that this case is likely to be appealed.

10.2.1 Capacity to make decisions about family or personal relationships

The court has no jurisdiction to intervene in disputes about family or personal relationships unless it is established that the person is incapable of making a decision about the matter in issue. Capacity to make a decision was considered in two medical treatment cases (described in section 12.3.1), first *Re C (Adult: Refusal of Medical Treatment)*[11] and later refined in *Re MB (Medical Treatment)*.[12] The latter case established a two-stage test of capacity to make a decision, in which in order to be deemed competent the person must be able to both:

- understand and retain the information relevant to the decision in question, especially as to the likely consequences, and
- use that information and weigh it in the balance as part of the process of arriving at a decision.

The test of capacity set out in the case *Re MB* was in the context of capacity to consent to or refuse medical treatment.

Nevertheless, the Official Solicitor's view, which was endorsed by the court, is that the test can be used for a wide range of decisions.[13] This is, therefore, the relevant test to apply in determining whether an individual has capacity to make decisions concerning family and personal relationships.

10.3 Sexual relationships

Deciding to enter into a sexual relationship with another individual is a personal decision which does not generally require any formal contract or test of capacity. Men and women can give legal consent to either opposite or same sex relationships at the age of 16.[14] Relationships can be of any duration and of varying degrees of intensity and commitment. Sexual relationships are personal in nature, which means that it is entirely for the individuals involved to decide whether or not to embark upon them. Even the courts cannot make that decision on behalf of incapacitated people who are over 16 but, nevertheless, society has obligations to ensure that their choice is voluntary.

10.3.1 Capacity to consent to sexual relationships

Since there is no specific test designed to cover consent to sexual relations in the context of the civil law concerning a person's private rights, where a test of capacity is needed the general two-stage test of capacity set out in the case of *Re MB* would be the relevant one (see section 10.2.1). This says that the person must be able to understand and retain information about what is involved and be able to weigh the information in the balance to arrive at a choice. It is also important that the particular circumstances of the individuals involved are taken into account. (Some suggested factors for assessment are listed below.) For example, it is essential to consider whether one person is in a position of power which influences the ability of the other to consent in an unpressured way. As discussed in section 10.1, it should also be noted that different considerations apply in determining capacity to give valid consent in the context of the criminal law, and particularly where it is alleged that a sexual offence has taken place (see Chapter 11).

Relatives or carers may try to stop a relationship involving people with a learning disability because of concerns about pregnancy, risks of infection, moral objections to the existence of a sexual relationship, or opposition to possible future marriage and parenthood. Doctors may be asked to give a view about the appropriateness of two people embarking on a close relationship and there may be concern about the ability of one or both parties to give valid consent to sexual intercourse. It is important that each party is seen privately and assessed individually before doctors advise on the person's capacity. Every attempt must be made to provide individuals with the information they require to be able to make a decision as to whether or not to have a sexual relationship. For example, they may need advice about contraception or other risks of intercourse. The following factors may be relevant to an assessment of individuals' capacity to consent to sexual relations:

- their understanding of what is involved in sexual intercourse
- their knowledge (at a basic level) of the risks of pregnancy and sexually transmitted diseases
- the kind of relationship they have (for example, if there is a power imbalance)
- the pleasure (or otherwise) which they experience in the relationship.

A lack of capacity to consent formally to sexual relations does not necessarily mean that the relationship should be prevented or discouraged, as long as the individuals appear willing and content for it to continue. If, however, there are signs that either person is being sexually abused or exploited, the matter should be immediately reported to the police so the protection given by the criminal law can be brought into effect (see Chapter 11). If, on the other hand, it is felt that the individuals enjoy and benefit from a non-abusive sexual relationship, consideration must be given to promoting their best interests in terms of providing contraception, and protection from infection (see section 12.4 on treatment of adults who lack capacity to consent). In some cases, for example, the possibility of offering sterilisation may be appropriate if this seems to be in the best interests of the patient.

10.4 Capacity to consent to marriage

People with mental illness or learning disability may marry if they have a broad understanding of what marriage is. The marriage ceremony requires both parties to enter into a contract. Capacity to do this was considered by the courts in a number of cases in the 1870s and 1880s. In the case of *Hunter v Edney*,[15] Sir James Hannen made the following statement about marriage, distinguishing between marriage and the wedding ceremony itself. He said: "The question which I have to determine is not whether she was aware that she was going through the ceremony of marriage, but whether she was capable of understanding the nature of the contract she was entering into". In order to understand the marriage contract, the person must be free from the influence of any "morbid delusions".

10.4.1 Level of understanding required for marriage

The degree of understanding required in order to have capacity to enter into the marriage contract was considered in the case of *Durham v Durham* in which Sir James Hannen also said "the contract of marriage is a very simple one which does not require a high degree of intelligence to understand. It is an engagement between a man and a woman to live together, and love one another as husband and wife, to the exclusion of all others."[16]

In the more recent case of *In the Estate of Park, Park v Park*[17] the level of understanding was expressed as a broad understanding of "the duties and responsibilities normally entailing to a marriage". In this case, Robert Park was undoubtedly suffering from dementia when he married Wyn Hughes, who worked as a cashier at his London club. He made a new will on his wedding day, making modest provision for his new wife. He died a few weeks later, before the marriage was consummated. In the action which followed, a jury found he was not of sound mind, memory and understanding when he executed the will, and probate was refused. This rendered him intestate and further litigation ensued as to whether he had capacity to consent to the marriage which had revoked his earlier will. The Court of Appeal held that Mr Park had the capacity to enter into a valid and binding marriage. He therefore died intestate and his widow was entitled to a substantial portion of his estate.

10.4.2 The effect of mental disorder

Under the Matrimonial Causes Act 1973 a marriage is voidable (that is, it can be annulled at the request of one of the parties) if at the time of marriage either party, although capable of giving valid consent, was suffering (whether continuously or intermittently) from mental disorder of such a kind or to such an extent as to be unfitted to marriage.[18] The mental disorder (for definition, see section 4.2.2) may be of the petitioner or the respondent.

To succeed in proving that a marriage is voidable, the petitioner must show that the person's mental disorder made him or her incapable of living in a married state and carrying out the duties and obligations of marriage. Merely being difficult to live with will not make a person unfitted to marriage, however.[19] This provision of the Matrimonial Causes Act is not strictly a "capacity test".

Proceedings must be started within 3 years of the marriage, although the court may give leave for proceedings to be instituted at a later date. The court may not grant a decree in the case of a voidable marriage if the petitioner, knowing it was open to him or her to have the marriage avoided, had acted in such a way that the respondent reasonably believed an annulment would not be sought and it would be unjust to grant a decree (for example, in a marriage for companionship only). A doctor asked to give an opinion about such an application should consult with those who know the party who is alleged to be mentally disordered and who have professional experience of the mental disorder.

10.4.3 What objections can be raised to a proposed marriage?

Sometimes a relative or carer of a person with marginal capacity is concerned about a proposed marriage. There are a number of ways in which an objection to a pending marriage can be made. A person can:

- dissent from the publication of banns in the case of a church wedding
- enter a caveat against the granting of a special or common licence
- enter a caveat with a superintendent registrar or the Registrar General (in the case of register office or other civil weddings).

If a caveat is entered, this puts the registrar or clergyman on notice and creates a requirement to investigate and enquire into the capacity of both parties to marry. The burden of proof of lack of capacity falls on the person seeking to oppose the marriage. The registrar may ask for a doctor's report or a report from a social worker, a psychologist, or other person who can give information about the ability of the parties to understand the contract of marriage. The tests to be applied are those stated above (section 10.4) and it is important that a full consultation with all relevant people takes place. Any opinion should be based on a sound knowledge of the person, his or her way of life and any relevant religious or cultural facts. It is not necessary for the person to appreciate or consider every aspect of a marital relationship (see section 10.4.1).

When one or both parties proposing to marry has a learning disability it may be important to suggest counselling and advice about the practical aspects of marriage including financial, housing and legal matters. Information and advice about sexuality and sexual relations, including contraception, may be useful and should be made available. A judgment about the person's capacity to understand the responsibilities of parenthood may also be relevant here. For example, additional support may be needed to avoid the possibility of future proceedings under the Children Act 1989 resulting in a child being removed from the person's care.

10.4.4 Implications of marriage

As discussed in section 10.4.1 above, the level of understanding required for marriage is less than that required for some other decisions or transactions. Since the status of marriage affects other matters, such as financial affairs and rights to property, subsequent arrangements may need to be made for a person who lacks capacity to manage these affairs (see Chapter 4). In particular, marriage revokes any existing will made by either of the parties. If one person lacks testamentary capacity (see section 5.2) an application may need to be made to the Court of Protection for a statutory will to be made on the person's behalf[20] (see section 5.7).

10.5 Capacity to separate or divorce

There are no reported court decisions concerning the capacity required to separate or divorce except in the Ontario Court[21] (such decisions are regarded as persuasive but not binding on UK courts). Mr and Mrs Calvert married in 1979, having signed a pre-marriage contract which said that any property owned by one of the parties at the date of the agreement would not be a family asset. Mrs Calvert managed a clothes shop and Mr Calvert owned a substantial farm in Ontario. Each of them had a grown-up child from a previous marriage. Nine years later Mr Calvert sold the farm for a small fortune. Despite his enormous wealth, he paid his wife a minimal allowance and begrudged the small gifts she sent to her daughter and grandchildren. In 1993, Mrs Calvert began to show signs of the early stages of Alzheimer's disease. A few months later, however, she made her own arrangements to visit her daughter in Calgary and she travelled alone. She never returned to her husband and instructed a lawyer to start divorce proceedings. Mr Calvert contended that his wife did not have capacity to form the intention to separate from him and thus was not entitled to any financial settlement. Relying on *In the Estate of Park, Park v Park* (see section 10.4.1) the Ontario Court recognised the varying levels of capacity required to make different decisions and gave separate consideration to the three levels of capacity relevant to that case: capacity to separate, capacity to divorce, and capacity to instruct counsel in connection with the divorce. The judge held as follows:

> Separation is the simplest act requiring the lowest level of understanding. A person has to know with whom he or she does or does not want to live. Divorce, while still simple, requires a bit more understanding. It requires the desire to remain separate and to be no longer married to one's spouse. It is the undoing of the contract of

marriage. ... If marriage is simple, divorce must be equally simple ... the mental capacity required for divorce is the same as required for entering into a marriage. ... The capacity to instruct counsel involves the ability to understand financial and legal issues. This puts it significantly higher on the competence hierarchy. ... While Mrs Calvert may have lacked the ability to instruct counsel, that did not mean she could not make the basic personal decision to separate and divorce.[22]

Chapter 7 provides further details on capacity to litigate and on the appointment of a "litigation friend" or "next friend" to act on behalf of people involved in legal proceedings (such as divorce proceedings) who lack capacity to instruct a legal representative. Further advice about capacity to instruct a solicitor is given in section 2.1.

10.6 Conclusion

It is important to remember the rights of people with a disability or illness when considering their ability to make their own decisions. As noted above, the United Nations Declaration of Human Rights states that all adults are of equal value and have a right to the same freedoms. One of these rights for adults is the right to express their sexuality and to participate in family life.

References and notes

1   European Convention on Human Rights, Article 8.
2   Ibid: Article 12.
3   See R v Jenkins (2000) (Unreported) described in: Winchester R. Pressure builds to revamp consent laws in wake of failed rape charge. *Community Care* 2000; **3–9 Feb**:10–11. In this case, the prosecution of a care worker accused of raping a woman with severe learning disabilities collapsed after the judge accepted the interpretation of consent ("submitting to animal instincts") used in the out-dated case of R v Fletcher (1866) LR 1 CCR; this was in preference to the evidence of an expert witness who had assessed that the complainant lacked capacity to consent to sexual relations. The expert witness had based her assessment on the guidance in the 1995 edition of this book, which the judge ruled was wrong in the context of criminal proceedings. However, the public outrage about this case gave added impetus to the need for reform of the criminal law on sexual offences contained in the Sexual Offences Bill, which when implemented, will introduce a new definition of consent (see Chapter 11).

4   Children Act 1989, s1.
5   Children Act 1989, s8.
6   Re S (Adult Patient: Jurisdiction)[1995] 1 FLR 302.
7   Re S (Hospital Patient: Court's Jurisdiction)[1995] 3 All ER 290.
8   See for example: Re D-R (Contact: Mentally Incapacitated Adult)[1999] 2 FCR 49.
9   Re F (Adult: Court's jurisdiction)[2000] 2 FLR 512.
10 Re S (Adult patient) (Inherent Jurisdiction: Family Life) [2003] 1 FLR 292: 306.
11 Re C (Adult: Refusal of Medical Treatment) [1994] 1 All ER 819.
12 Re MB (Medical Treatment) [1997] 2 FLR 426: 437.
13 Practice Note (Official Solicitor: Declaratory Proceedings) [2001] 2 FLR 158, paragraph 7[1]. The Practice Note is set out at Appendix C.
14 Sexual Offences (Amendment) Act 2000, s1.
15 Hunter v Edney (1885) 10 PD 93.
16 Durham v Durham (1885) 10 PD 80.
17 In the Estate of Park, Park v Park [1954] P 112.
18 Matrimonial Causes Act 1973, s11–13.
19 Bennett v Bennett [1969] 1 WLR 430.
20 Re Davey (Deceased) [1980] 3 All ER 342.
21 Calvert (Litigation Guardian) v Calvert (1997) 32 OR (3d) 281.
22 Ibid: 293f, 294g and 298e–g.

11 Capacity to consent: the criminal law and sexual offences

This chapter deals with the approach of the criminal law towards sexual behaviour and people who are vulnerable because of mental disability. The primary focus of the criminal law is upon non-consensual conduct; however, it is recognised that persons with mental disabilities have an equal right to express their sexuality and to form relationships commensurate with their ability to give consent[1] (see Chapter 10). The role of the law is to police the line between the legitimate right of all adult persons to engage in sexual relationships and the need to protect the vulnerable from exploitation and abuse.

11.1 Proposed changes to the law

The law relating to sexual offences has evolved in piecemeal and unsatisfactory fashion, described in a Home Office Consultation paper as a "patchwork quilt of provisions ancient and modern".[2] Following lengthy consultation, the Sexual Offences Bill was introduced. It was put before the House of Lords on 28 January 2003.[3] The Bill seeks to clarify the crucial issue of "consent": it contains a general definition of the term, as well as listing a series of situations where consent would be presumed to be absent (see section 11.1.1). It also re-defines the offences to reflect increased public awareness and changes in sexual conduct.

The Bill contains specific revisions in connection with vulnerable groups such as people with mental disability. Its general definition of consent requires a person to have the "capacity" to choose whether to agree to sexual activity, although there is no general definition of "capacity" in the Bill. If consent is absent, the defendant's honest but unreasonable belief that it is present will no longer prevent a finding of guilt. The Bill also creates specific offences against people with a mental disorder or a learning disability, including a category of offences specific to care workers.

At the time of writing, the Bill was still being considered in Parliament. In the following sections, therefore, a description is given of both the provisions of law in effect at the time of writing and the changes proposed in the Sexual Offences Bill as amended in the House of Lords. At the time of writing it was not clear if and when the Bill would become law or when its provisions would be implemented. It must also be noted that the Bill may change during its remaining parliamentary stages and it cannot be assumed that the information provided here will be the same as in the Act itself – if and when finally approved. Those requiring up-to-date information on the law on sexual offences should consult the BMA website (http://www.bma.org.uk/ethics).

11.1.1 Consent and mental capacity

Law in effect at September 2003

Victims of sexual abuse who lack mental capacity are described in the current legislation in obsolete and offensive fashion as "defective". This is defined as a "state of incomplete development of mind which includes severe impairment of intelligence and social functioning" when measured against the standard of "normal persons".[4]

Any professional considering what action to take concerning the possible commission of an offence against a vulnerable person will need to be aware of the statutory difference in the protection afforded depending upon what offence is alleged, particularly with regard to the issue of consent. The most common offences that will arise in connection with the abuse of people with mental disabilities will be indecent assault and rape. In law, a person lacking in mental capacity cannot give consent to what would otherwise be an indecent assault, but that person can consent to sexual intercourse. Therefore, in rape cases the prosecution must show that the victim did not consent, or was not capable of consenting, whereas with sexual assault it need only be proved that the sexual activity took place and that the victim has a mental disability amounting to a lack of capacity. This anomaly means that the more serious offence of rape is often more difficult to prove.

Proposals under the Sexual Offences Bill

A person consents if he or she agrees by choice and has the freedom and capacity to make that choice, although there is no general definition of "capacity" in the Bill. Where the defendant intentionally deceived the victim as to the nature or purpose of the relevant act, or intentionally induced the complainant to consent to it by impersonating someone known personally to the complainant, consent will conclusively be presumed to be absent. A series of situations are also set out where it will be presumed that no consent exists unless evidence is adduced to raise an issue to the contrary. These include situations of violence, fear of violence, or unlawful detention, and situations where the complainant had been asleep or unconscious or unable to communicate whether they consented due to physical disability.

11.1.2 Rape

Law in effect at September 2003

Rape is sexual intercourse, whether vaginal or anal, with a complainant without his or her consent.[5] To be guilty of rape the perpetrator must know that the person does not consent or must be reckless as to whether consent is given. The burden of proving the absence of consent lies upon the prosecution.

It is important to bear in mind the following general principles, which apply in all cases where rape is alleged, whatever the capacity of the complainant.

- The vital ingredients of the offence are sexual intercourse[6] and lack of consent.
- The use of force is not required.
- The victim's consent may be vitiated by threat, duress, or inculcation of fear.
- Mere submission does not equate to consent although the dividing line may on occasion be difficult to draw.[7]

Where a complainant is vulnerable because of extreme youth or lack of mental capacity, the law of rape currently provides no extra statutory protection. Where a complainant is capable of sexual feeling it cannot necessarily be presumed that lack of consent will automatically be shown by reason of mental incapacity.[8] Although a complainant's lack of understanding may be relevant as to whether consent was in fact given, this factor will generally not absolve the prosecution of their duty of proof.

Where a complainant is able to give evidence the jury will accordingly have to decide whether she or he did in fact consent whatever their difficulties. A particular problem may arise where the complainant is not capable of giving a lucid or coherent account of events since expert evidence of limited mental age, social functioning or intellectual impairment will not necessarily prove lack of consent apart from in the most extreme cases.

The prosecution in these cases may currently have to grasp the nettle and seek a conviction for an alternative lesser offence.[9] The consequence may be that a perpetrator faces on conviction a markedly lower sentence than his behaviour might otherwise justify.

Proposals under the Sexual Offences Bill

There are substantial alterations to the ingredients of the offence. The offence will be committed, in addition to the current forms of rape, by non-consensual penetration of the mouth. In the case of victims under 13 years of age, there will be no need to prove lack of consent. For victims over 13 years of age, the definition of consent set out above will apply, as will the presumptions against consent in certain situations, and any mistaken belief in consent by the defendant must be reasonable (see section 11.1.1). The proposed revisions therefore provide extra protection for victims who are vulnerable because of mental disability or extreme youth.

11.1.3 Indecent assault

Law in effect at September 2003

Indecent assault is defined as an unwanted touching or interference with a person in "circumstances of indecency". It may involve either overt sexual interference or less intimate contact accompanied by words or actions of a sexual nature. Although consent – as in rape – will be a defence, the law makes the important provision that where the person touched is "defective" then that consent cannot normally be given as a matter of law,[10] unless the perpetrator establishes he neither knew nor had reason to suspect the victim's condition.

Proposals under the Sexual Offences Bill

Indecent assault is replaced with several different offences: assault by penetration (with a separate offence relating to child victims), sexual assault (or sexual assault on a child under 13), and causing a person to engage in sexual activity without consent (or causing or inciting a child under 13 to engage in sexual activity). The Bill deals with consent for indecent assault in the same way as consent for rape (see section 11.1.2 above).

11.1.4 Other sexual offences against people with learning disabilities

Law in effect at September 2003

There are an additional five measures contained in the Sexual Offences Act 1956 aimed at the protection of women with severe learning disabilities, namely the prohibition on:

- sexual intercourse with a woman who is a "defective" (s7)
- the procuring of a woman who is a "defective" to have sexual intercourse (s9)
- the taking of a "defective" from her parent or guardian for the purpose of sexual intercourse (s21)
- allowing premises to be used by a "defective" for the purpose of unlawful sexual intercourse (s27)
- encouraging prostitution by a "defective" (s29).

In all of these offences it is a common defence for the accused to show that he did not know nor had any reason to suspect that the person concerned was a "defective".

Proposals under the Sexual Offences Bill

The above offences are replaced with new offences specific to victims with a mental disorder or learning disability. The offences are committed by sexual activity with or in the presence or view of someone who is unable to refuse because they are suffering from mental disorder or learning disability, or by intentionally causing or inciting such a person to engage in sexual activity. It must be the case that the defendant knows, or could reasonably be expected to know, of the victim's condition and that this is likely to make them unable to refuse. A separate group of clauses create offences where the same situations are brought about by inducement, threat or deception.

Where some capacity to consent exists there may still be the potential for exploitation. Even where a potentially vulnerable individual fully understands and consents to a sexual relationship there may be grounds for the criminal law to intervene for public policy reasons should that person be under the professional care of the other.

A final group of offences in the Bill can be committed only by "care workers". This term is defined to include workers in NHS bodies, independent medical agencies, care homes, community homes, voluntary homes, and children's homes, independent clinics, and independent hospitals, who have had or are likely to have regular face-to-face contact with the victim in the course of their employment. It also includes those who, whether or not in the course of employment, provide care, assistance, or services to the victim in connection with the victim's learning disability or mental disorder, if as such they have had or are likely to have regular face-to-face contact with the victim.

11.2 Giving evidence in court

11.2.1 Assisting the vulnerable witness

Even if a vulnerable person is able to provide a witness statement as to an alleged assault upon him or her, giving evidence to a court may be more difficult. The legal process can be intimidating or confusing enough to potential witnesses who do not lack capacity. For someone with learning disabilities or other mental disorder it may be practically impossible. For such a witness the terms used by lawyers and the purpose of specific questions may cause such bewilderment that the ends of justice may be difficult to achieve.

The need to offer effective assistance in giving evidence to those who may be particularly vulnerable has been addressed in Part II of the Youth Justice and Criminal Evidence Act 1999. A lack of ability to understand and communicate may in due course be met by the making of a "special measures direction". This will enable the witness to receive assistance from an intermediary in explaining questions and communicating answers "so far as is necessary to enable them to be understood by the witness or person in question".[11]

A witness is eligible for this assistance[12] if she or he suffers from mental disorder within the meaning of mental health legislation (currently the Mental Health Act 1983) or otherwise has "significant impairment of intelligence and social functioning". The purpose of providing the assistance is to preserve the "quality" of the witness' evidence in terms of its "completeness, coherence and accuracy".[13]

The presence in court of the alleged abuser may provide a powerful disincentive for a vulnerable witness to give an account of what took place. Legislation now permits the giving of evidence by pre-recorded video tape and cross-examination via a video link, thereby avoiding the need for direct confrontation of complainant and accused.[14] Formerly these arrangements existed only in respect of prosecutions for sexual offences where the alleged victim was under 17 years of age when the tape was recorded.[15]

11.2.2 The absent witness

At present if a witness is unable to give evidence consideration may be given to having his or her witness statement read to the court instead.[16] This is however subject to strict rules. The witness must be "unfit to attend as a witness" by reason of "bodily or mental condition" or, having made the statement to a person investigating an offence, be now too afraid to give oral evidence.

Having regard to the fact that the witness could not then be cross-examined the procedure is permitted only at the discretion of the trial judge who may rule that it would not be in the interests of justice to do so.

Whatever the difficulties a prosecution may in certain circumstances proceed in the absence of the complainant's evidence provided that "consent" is not the primary issue. In those circumstances it may be practically impossible to secure a conviction. Where a complainant's consent is not material, for example, in indecent assault cases given his or her status in law as a "defective" then the essential requirement will be evidence to prove that sexual touching or interference took place combined with proof of the condition of the complainant.

11.3 Conclusion

The rights of persons with mental disabilities to make their own decisions, to express their sexuality and to participate as fully as possible in family life remain profoundly important. Whether the criminal law appears to strike the correct balance between protection of vulnerable people on the one hand, and an unduly paternalistic and authoritarian stance upon the other, will doubtless depend upon the circumstances of each individual case.

It is to be hoped nonetheless that the proposed changes in the law will make the boundaries clearer and assist in the protection of people with mental disabilities and the prosecution of those who would exploit their vulnerability.

References and notes

1 The right to private life, of which intimate sexual activity forms a part, is protected by Article 8 of the European Convention on Human Rights.
2 Home Office. *Setting the boundaries: reforming the law on sex offences.* London: The Stationery Office, 2000: iii.
3 Sexual Offences Bill, HL Bill 26. See also: Law Commission, *Consent in sex offences: A report to the Home Office Sex Offences Review.* London: Law Commission, 2000.
4 Sexual Offences Act 1956, s45. See: R v Hall (1988) 86 Cr. App. R 159.
5 Sexual Offences Act 1956 as amended by the Criminal Justice and Public Order Act 1994, s1(2a).
6 Partial penetration will suffice.
7 See: R v Olugboja [1981] 3 WLR 585:585–593.
8 See: the old case of R v Fletcher (1866) LR 1 CCR, which refers crudely to the "animal instincts" of the complainant. The controversial failure of the prosecution in R v Jenkins (2000) (unreported) – a case withdrawn from the jury at the Central Criminal Court where this authority was recited with approval – shows that this approach is still liable to be regarded as correct. However different judges may take different views as to the effect of learning disability in any particular case before them. Other old cases,

such as those of R v Barratt (1873) LR 2 CCR 81 and R v Pressy (1867) 10 Cox 635 suggest a measure of discretion in allowing a case to go to a jury.

9   For example under s7(1) Sexual Offences Act 1956, that is having "unlawful sexual intercourse with a woman who is a defective".

10 Sexual Offences Act, s14(4) (woman), s15(3) (man). Consent is also unavailable as a defence where the victim is under 16.

11 Youth Justice and Criminal Evidence Act 1999, s29(2). Only in force regarding power to make Rules of the Court.

12 Ibid: s16(2).

13 Ibid: s16(1)(b), (5).

14 Ibid: s24, s27.

15 Criminal Justice Act 1988 (now repealed), s32A(7).

16 Criminal Justice Act 1988, s23(1)–(3).

12 Capacity to consent to and refuse medical treatment

12.1 Medical procedures

This chapter deals with the capacity of adult patients to consent and refuse consent to medical procedures. "Medical procedures" means examination, diagnostic tests, and medical or nursing interventions aimed at alleviating a medical condition or preventing its deterioration. Therapies designed to rehabilitate patients are also included in this definition. Medical research and innovative treatments are considered in Chapter 13.

12.2 The need for patient consent

In most cases, health professionals cannot legally examine or treat any adult without his or her valid consent. No-one else (not even a husband or wife or other close relative) can give or withhold consent to medical treatment on behalf of another adult.

In general, it is unlawful and unethical to treat a person who is capable of understanding and willing to know, without first explaining the nature of the procedure, its purpose and implications, and obtaining that person's agreement.[1] Every effort must be made to explain these issues in terms the patient can understand, offering appropriate support and other aids to communication. Some people consent to treatment while choosing not to be told the full details of their diagnosis or treatment. Their "uninformed" consent is nevertheless valid so long as they had the option of receiving more information. People who refuse information must still be provided with basic information, since without this they cannot make a valid choice to delegate responsibility for treatment decisions to the doctor. The amount of basic information needed depends upon the individual circumstances, the severity of the condition, and the risks associated with the treatment. Doctors must seek to strike a balance between giving the patient sufficient information for a valid decision, and respecting the patient's wish not to know.

An exception is treatment provided under mental health legislation which authorises assessment of individuals, their admission to hospital and, if necessary, treatment for a mental disorder without their consent. The treatment provisions of the Mental Health Act 1983 (which was under review at the time of writing) are not discussed in detail in this book since they are well covered elsewhere.[2] While some people who lack capacity to consent may need compulsory treatment for mental disorder under the provisions of mental health legislation, many people accept treatment without any resistance, even though they may not understand the nature and purpose of the treatment given.

The legal basis for providing treatment and restricting the free movement of incapacitated patients was challenged in the *Bournewood* case[3] concerning the "detention" in hospital of a 48-year-old man. This patient, known as L, suffered from autism with other complex disabilities, resulting in an inability to communicate or express preferences. After being a patient in Bournewood Hospital for 30 years he went to live with a family of carers under an adult placement scheme where he settled well. One day, while at the local day centre, L became agitated and distressed. His carers could not be contacted so he was taken to the local accident and emergency department, from where he was admitted to Bournewood Hospital. Despite requests from his carers for him to return home, he remained an in-patient. Had he attempted to leave, his consultant made clear that he would have been detained under the Mental Health Act 1983. A case was taken to court on L's behalf, challenging his continued "detention" and treatment in hospital. The House of Lords ultimately determined that compliant incapacitated patients can be treated for mental disorder without their consent under common law, outside the provisions of the 1983 Act, on the basis that they neither resist nor refuse treatment and compulsion is therefore unnecessary. The case highlighted, however, that such patients do not benefit from the safeguards offered to detained patients to challenge their detention and treatment under mental health legislation.

This situation was described by Lord Steyn as "an indefensible gap in our mental health law".[4] The government made a commitment to fill that gap, in particular to ensure compliance with Article 5 of the European Convention on Human Rights, by introducing further safeguards in mental health legislation against inappropriate treatment or detention of compliant incapacitated patients.[5] Even when those changes are introduced, however, patients who lack capacity to consent to treatment for mental disorder, and who do not resist that treatment, will continue to be treated informally under the provisions of the common law described in this chapter, in the same way as those requiring treatment for physical disorders.

12.3 Capacity to consent to medical procedures

As discussed in Part IV of this book, assessing capacity is a time-consuming exercise and some measures can enhance the perceived capacity of the person being assessed and maximise his or her ability to communicate (see also section 2.3 on optimising the conditions for assessment of capacity). The legal presumption of capacity until the contrary is shown is important (see Part II). Assessing capacity to consent to medical treatment is somewhat different to other capacity assessments since the assessor may also be the person proposing the treatment. If the procedure proposed is a risky one or involves innovative techniques, or if there is a divergence of opinion as to its benefits for the patient, additional safeguards are likely to be needed (see also Chapter 13 on research).

12.3.1 Consent to treatment and other procedures

The assessment of an adult patient's capacity to make a decision about his or her own medical treatment is a matter for clinical judgment guided by professional practice and subject to legal requirements. It is the personal responsibility of any doctor proposing to treat a patient to judge whether the patient has the capacity to give a valid consent. The doctor has a duty to give the patient an account in simple terms of the benefits and risks of the proposed treatment and explain the principal alternatives to it. Two cases have been particularly significant in setting out the test of capacity required to make a decision about medical treatment. The first case of *Re C (Adult: Refusal of Medical Treatment)*[6] considered whether a schizophrenic patient detained in a high security hospital had capacity to refuse consent to the amputation of his gangrenous foot. The High Court held that an adult has capacity to consent to (or refuse consent to) medical treatment, if he or she can:

- understand and retain the information relevant to the decision in question
- believe that information, and
- weigh that information in the balance to arrive at a choice.

The second case *Re MB (Medical Treatment)*[7] concerned a pregnant woman's refusal to consent to the medical procedures necessary for a Caesarean section (specifically venepuncture) because of her phobia to needles. The Court of Appeal noted the presumption of capacity and confirmed that a competent woman may, for religious or other reasons, for rational or irrational reasons, or for no reason at all, choose not to have medical intervention, even though the consequences may be death or serious handicap of the child she bears, or her own death. The Court held that a person lacks capacity if some impairment or disturbance of mental functioning renders the person unable to make a decision whether to consent to or refuse treatment. The inability to make a decision occurs when:

- the patient is unable to comprehend and retain the information which is material to the decision, especially as to the consequences of having or not having the treatment in question; or
- the patient is unable to use the information and weigh it in the balance as part of the process of arriving at a decision.

The Court found that MB's fear of needles induced such panic that "... at that moment the needle or mask dominated her thinking and made her quite unable to consider anything else".[8] She therefore lacked the necessary capacity to make the decision to consent to or refuse treatment which made her refusal ineffective.

The principles that arise from these and other legal cases are that, in order to demonstrate capacity, individuals should be able to:

- understand in simple language what the medical treatment is, its nature and purpose, and why it is being proposed
- understand its principal benefits, risks, and alternatives
- understand in broad terms what will be the consequences of not receiving the proposed treatment
- retain the information for long enough to use it and weigh it in the balance in order to arrive at a decision.

In order for the consent to be valid, the patient must be able to make a free choice (that is to say free from pressure – see section 12.3.2). All assessments of an individual's capacity should be fully recorded in the patient's medical notes.

12.3.2 Refusal of medical procedures

Competent adults have a clear right to refuse medical diagnostic procedures or treatment for reasons which are "rational, irrational or for no reason". This principle was established in the case of *Sidaway v Board of Governors of the Bethlem Royal Hospital and Maudsley Hospital*[9] and upheld in *Re MB* (see section 12.3.1). The person's capacity to refuse in a valid manner must be assessed in relation to the specific treatment proposed and the gravity of the decision to be made. It is irrelevant whether refusal is contrary to the views of most other people if it is broadly consistent with the individual's own value system.

The principle that an adult patient has the right to refuse treatment as long as he or she has been properly informed of the implications and can make a free choice was affirmed by the Court of Appeal in the case of *Re T (Adult: Refusal of Treatment)*.[10] That case concerned a 20-year-old woman who was injured in a road traffic accident when she was 34 weeks pregnant. She had been brought up as a Jehovah's Witness and on admission to hospital refused a blood transfusion after having spent a period of time alone with her mother. T gave birth to a stillborn child after which her condition became critical. Her father and boyfriend applied for a court declaration that it would not be unlawful to administer a transfusion without her consent.

The Court of Appeal held that for such a refusal to be valid, doctors had to be satisfied that the patient's capacity to decide had not been diminished by illness, medication, false assumptions, or misinformation, or that the patient's will had not been overborne by another's influence. In T's situation it was held that the effect of her condition, together with misinformation and her mother's influence, rendered her refusal of consent ineffective.

What is important about this case, notwithstanding the outcome for the individual patient, is the general affirmation of a patient's right, properly exercised, to refuse medical treatment. Lady Justice Butler Sloss confirmed that:

> A man or woman of full age and sound understanding may choose to reject medical advice and medical or surgical treatment either partially or in its entirety. A decision to refuse medical treatment by a patient capable of making the decision does not have to be sensible, rational or well considered.[11]

A doctor's legal duties in relation to a patient's refusal of treatment were discussed in the same case when the Master of the Rolls stated:

> Doctors faced with a refusal of consent have to give very careful and detailed consideration to the patient's capacity to decide at the time when the decision was made. It may not be the simple case of the patient having no capacity because, for example, at that time he had hallucinations. It may be the more difficult case of a temporarily reduced capacity at the time when his decision was made. What matters is that the doctors should consider whether at that time he had a capacity which was commensurate with the gravity of the decision which he purported to make. The more serious the decision, the greater the capacity required. If the patient had the requisite capacity, they are bound by his decision. If not, they are free to treat him in what they believe to be his best interests.[12]

The judge recommended that in cases of uncertainty doctors seek a declaration from the courts as to the lawfulness of treatment.

If an individual appears to be choosing an option which is not only contradictory to that most people would choose, but also appears to contradict that individual's previously expressed attitudes, health professionals would be justified in questioning in greater detail that individual's capacity to make a valid refusal in order to investigate the possibility of a depressive illness or a delusional state or the effect of personality disorder. One example is the case involving the "moors murderer" Ian Brady, who had decided to starve himself to death and applied to court to challenge the decision of Ashworth Hospital to feed him forcibly. The judge held that:

> ... notwithstanding the fact that he is a man of well above average intelligence, he has engaged in his battle of wills in such a way that, as a result of his severe personality disorder, he has eschewed the weighing of information and the balancing of risks and needs to such an extent that ... his decisions on food refusal and force feeding have been incapacitated. As a result, the doctors have been legally empowered to supply medical treatment in his best interests.[13]

In such cases, a specialist psychiatric opinion may be required. Practical aspects of assessment of capacity are discussed in more detail in Part IV of this book.

12.4 Treatment of adults lacking capacity to consent

If an adult patient temporarily or permanently lacks capacity to consent to medical treatment no other person can consent to medical treatment on the patient's behalf. Some forms of medical treatment are lawful, however, even in the absence of the patient's consent. The legal basis for carrying out a medical procedure in such cases is that the procedures are "necessary".

12.4.1 The concept of necessity

The concept of "necessity" permitting doctors to provide treatment without obtaining the patient's consent was explained in the House of Lords in *Re F (Mental Patient:*

Sterilisation). This was the first case in which the courts were asked to declare that sterilisation for non-therapeutic purposes was not unlawful. Their Lordships held that for treatment to be justified:

> ... not only (1) must there be a necessity to act when it is not practicable to communicate with the assisted person, but also (2) the action taken must be such as a reasonable person would in all the circumstances take, acting in the best interests of the assisted person.[14]

Although it is often assumed that the doctrine of necessity applies only to emergency situations, this is not the case. As defined by the Law Lords in *Re F (Mental Patient: Sterilisation)*, the doctrine of necessity permits:

> ... action properly taken to preserve the life, health or well-being of the assisted person [which] may well transcend such measures as surgical operations or substantial medical treatment and may extend to include such humdrum matters as routine medical or dental treatment, even simple care such as dressing and undressing and putting to bed.[15]

Not only is a doctor able to give treatment to an incapacitated patient when it is clearly in that person's best interests, it is a common law duty to do so. Nevertheless, this still only applies to treatment carried out to ensure improvement or prevent deterioration in health or the steps required to prepare for recovery to become an option. If a person is now incapacitated, but is known to have objections to all or some treatment, doctors may not be justified in proceeding, even in an emergency (see section 12.5.2 on advance refusals). If the incapacity is temporary because of anaesthetic, sedation, intoxication, or temporary unconsciousness, doctors should not proceed beyond what is essential to preserve the person's life or prevent deterioration in health.

12.4.2 Best interests

The doctrine of necessity, which underpins treatment of people lacking capacity, is essentially made up of two components. First, there must be some necessity to act;

secondly, such action must be in the "best interests" of the person concerned (that is, that the expected benefits of a proposed treatment outweigh the burdens). Under the current law the second limb of the necessity concept means that a doctor who acts in accordance with an accepted body of medical opinion will generally be found to be acting in the best interests of the patient and will not be negligent in providing such treatment. The court has ruled, however, that best interests are not confined to best *medical* interests, but encompass broader emotional, social, and welfare considerations[16] and must take into account the patient's values and preferences when competent, their well-being, and quality of life, relationships with family or other carers, spiritual and religious welfare, and their own financial interests.

Where patients are competent and have access to information, they are the best judge of what is in their interests. Where patients lack capacity, the following factors are important in deciding what is in their best interests:

- the patient's own wishes and values (where these can be ascertained) including any advance statement (see section 12.5)
- clinical judgment about the effectiveness of the proposed treatment, particularly in relation to other options
- where there is more than one effective option, which option is the least restrictive of the patient's future choices
- the likelihood and extent of any degree of improvement in the patient's condition if treatment is provided
- the views of people close to the patient, especially close relatives, partners or carers about what the patient is likely to see as beneficial
- any knowledge of the patient's religious, cultural and other non-medical views that might have an impact on the patient's wishes.

12.4.3 Treatment safeguards and procedures

Treatment decisions can be divided into broad categories, some of which require the involvement of a court.

- For most low-level decisions, there should generally be agreement between health professionals, people close to the patient and the incapacitated person (in so far as he or she can express a view) as to treatment. Simple treatment or diagnostic options such as the taking of samples for anaemia or lithium levels, the provision of a mild analgesic for a headache, or antibiotics for an infection, in an otherwise fit person are uncontroversial. The decision can be taken by the clinician, the patient and people providing care.

- Some treatment decisions are so serious that the courts have said that each case should be brought before the courts for independent review. In particular, at the time of writing, all decisions involving the withdrawal of artificial hydration and nutrition from patients in a persistent vegetative state must be taken by the court,[17] although it is possible that this requirement may change. Other treatments currently requiring court decisions include non-therapeutic sterilisation,[18] and the harvesting of bone marrow.[19] In any case concerned with organ or tissue donation by an incapacitated person, it is essential that legal advice be obtained before the procedures are carried out.

The High Court has held that its involvement is not always necessary if a therapeutic operation will only have the incidental effect of sterilising a woman[20] or where termination of pregnancy is recommended.[21] There may be other medical procedures, however, which are likely to be so serious that they should be brought to the attention of the courts before they are carried out on an incapacitated patient. If doctors are in doubt, they should take advice from their professional, regulatory or indemnifying bodies, and may need to consult their lawyers.

Guidelines on the procedures to follow when a case is being taken to court were given by the courts in the case of *St George's Healthcare NHS Trust v S*.[22]

12.4.4 Views of relatives and others close to the patient

Although it is currently unnecessary and of no legal effect to ask relatives to sign consent forms on behalf of their adult relatives who lack capacity, it has, nevertheless, long been accepted medical practice to consult people close to the patient (bearing in mind the duty of confidentiality to the patient; see section 12.6) to help the medical team assess what the patient would have wanted and to determine the patient's best interests. In the case of *Re T (Adult: Refusal of Treatment)*[23] the court held that the views of relatives are important in so far as they reflect what the patient would have chosen if in a position to decide. While these views may not ultimately be determinative, they need to be factored into any decision about the patient's best interests. A balance must be sought between respecting the confidentiality rights of incapacitated people and judging what patients would wish to happen.

12.4.5 General principles

A number of general principles should be taken into account when considering the medical treatment of a patient lacking capacity. The patient's rights are described below.

- Liberty – patients should be free from interventions that inhibit liberty or the capacity to enjoy life unless such intervention is necessary to prevent a greater harm to the patient or to others. Treatment options should be the least restrictive effective option. Appropriate justification must be shown for the use of restraints and it is inappropriate for restrictive measures to be used as an alternative to adequate staffing levels.
- Autonomy – patients' autonomy should be promoted in a manner that is consistent with their needs and wishes.
- Dignity – patients should be treated with respect and courtesy, and their social and cultural values should be respected.
- Having their views taken into account – even when they are considered legally incapable of determining what happens.
- Privacy – patients should be free from any medical procedures unless there are good therapeutic reasons for them.
- Confidentiality – personal health information should be treated confidentially.
- Having their health needs met – these should be met as fully as practicable, while recognising that the availability of resources may limit treatment options.
- Being free from unfair discrimination – treatment options should be considered on the basis of the patient's need and

patients should not be treated differently solely because of the condition that gives rise to the incapacity.

- Having the views of people close to them taken into account – this applies even when they are not entitled in law to make decisions on behalf of the patient.

As a matter of good practice it is advisable to obtain a second opinion from another doctor in cases where a complex decision is contemplated, or where the benefits and burdens of treatment are finely balanced. This can both assure the doctor proposing to treat the patient that the patient does lack capacity to consent and that the treatment is in the patient's best interests. In its guidance *Withholding and withdrawing life-prolonging medical treatment*[25] the BMA provides examples of circumstances when it would be advisable to seek a second opinion.

For any serious procedure, the following steps are recommended as a useful guide:

- consider whether there are alternative ways of treating the patient, particularly equally effective measures which might be less invasive
- discuss the treatment with the healthcare team
- discuss the treatment with the patient in so far as this is possible
- consider any anticipatory statement of the patient's views (see section 12.5)
- consult relatives, carers or people close to the patient (see section 12.4.4)
- consult other appropriate professionals involved with the patient's care in the hospital or community
- consider the need to obtain a second opinion from a doctor skilled in the proposed treatment
- ensure that a record is made of the discussions.

12.4.6 Proposals for law reform

The Law Commission recommended a significant overhaul of the law governing the treatment of people who lack capacity to consent to medical treatment.[26] It recommended the introduction of a statutory authority for doctors to treat patients who are reasonably believed to lack capacity, provided it is reasonable for the doctor to provide the treatment and the treatment is in the best interests of the person. The Commission also recommended the introduction of new proxy decision making powers to allow consent for medical treatment to be given on behalf of an incapacitated adult. In June 2003, the government published a long-awaited Mental Incapacity Bill to reform the law along the lines recommended by the Law Commission. At the time of writing, the timescale for law reform was not known. Information about changes in the law relating to the provision of medical treatment for incapacitated adults will be put on the BMA website (http://www.bma.org.uk/ethics).

12.5 Capacity to make anticipatory decisions

Adults who are capable of making current medical decisions for themselves can, if properly informed of the implications and consequences, also make anticipatory decisions about their preferences for medical treatment at a later stage when their capacity may become impaired. Advance decisions cannot exceed those matters which a competent person can decide currently.

12.5.1 Advance statements

Advance statements are declarations whereby competent people make known their views on what should happen if they lose the capacity to make decisions for themselves. Advance statements can take a variety of forms ranging from general lists of life values and preferences, to specific requests or refusals of treatment. They can be written or oral. Their purpose is to provide a means for people to exercise autonomy by expressing an opinion in advance about future medical treatments. Individuals who are aware of a terminal illness or mental decline have often sought to discuss with their doctors how they wish to be treated. Advance statements enable a structured discussion and recording of the person's views to take place.

The test for capacity to make an advance statement about medical treatment is similar to that for capacity to make a contemporaneous medical decision. The treatment options, alternatives, and implications of them should be broadly understood. Individuals should also be aware that circumstances and medical science may develop in unforeseen ways in the interval before their advance statement becomes operative. Also if the statement concerns a positive consent to or claim for certain treatments, the person making the statement should be aware that doctors are not legally bound by such a consent. Doctors cannot be compelled to carry out treatments which are contrary to their clinical judgment. The BMA, together with the Royal Colleges and with the assistance of the Law Society, has published a detailed code of practice for health professionals on aspects of drafting, storage and implementation of advance statements, which summarises accepted practice and the law.[27] An information leaflet for patients has also been published by the Patients Association, summarising the issues that need to be taken into account in making an advance statement.[28]

12.5.2 Anticipatory refusals

It is clear in common law that competent, informed adults have a legal right to refuse medical procedures in advance.[29] A specific unambiguous and informed anticipatory refusal of treatment (also known as an advance directive or living will) is as valid as a contemporaneous decision and is therefore legally binding on health professionals so long as certain requirements are met. In case of uncertainty or dispute, courts may be asked to make a judgment as to the validity of the evidence of the person's intentions. A written, signed, and witnessed refusal is likely to be convincing evidence of a settled wish and should be presumed to be valid in the absence of any indication to the contrary.

In the Court of Appeal, in the case of *Re T (Adult: Refusal of Treatment)*[30] it was held that an advance refusal of treatment by an adult would be legally binding if it is:

- clearly established
- applicable to the current circumstances; and
- made without undue pressure from other people.

A clear and informed statement by a Jehovah's Witness refusing blood is an example of a potentially legally binding document. Any person making such a refusal should understand that the refusal of specific treatments may result in his or her death. In case of genuine doubt or ambiguity as to the individual's intention or capacity at the time of drafting, health professionals should adopt a "best interests" approach (see section 12.4.2) until clarification can be obtained.

Anticipatory refusals: General principles

The following principles emerge from the case law.

- An advance refusal of treatment is legally binding if the following four criteria apply:

  - the patient is an adult and was competent when the directive was made
  - the patient has been offered sufficient, accurate information to make an informed decision
  - the circumstances which have arisen are those which were envisaged by the patient, and
  - the patient was not subjected to undue influence in making the decision.

- Adults are presumed to be competent to make decisions, unless the contrary is shown. As with all decision making, the test of capacity to make an advance refusal of treatment is functional and the understanding required depends on the gravity of the decision.
- A refusal of treatment does not need to be a wise decision and the fact that a decision is contrary to what would be expected of the vast majority of adults does not affect its validity.

In cases of genuine doubt about the validity of an advance refusal, the presumption is in favour of providing life-saving treatment. Where there is doubt, and time permits, a declaration should be sought from a court.

Anybody, including health professionals and carers trained in providing treatment such as cardiopulmonary resuscitation, who knowingly provides treatment in the face of a valid advance refusal may be liable to legal action for battery or assault.

Advance "consent" or requests for treatment are not legally binding, although may be helpful in assessing a patient's likely wishes and preferences.

12.5.3 Scope of advance statements

Whatever wishes people express while competent should be given serious consideration. Nevertheless, people cannot authorise or refuse in advance procedures which they could not authorise or refuse contemporaneously. For example, they cannot authorise unlawful procedures, such as euthanasia, nor can they insist on futile or inappropriate treatment. The BMA also believes that advance statements refusing "basic care" and maintenance of comfort should not be binding on health professionals. Basic care includes the administration of medication or the performance of any procedure which is solely or primarily designed to provide comfort to the patient or alleviate that person's pain, symptoms, or distress.[31]

12.5.4 Proposals for law reform

There is currently no legislation covering advance decision making about medical treatment. In its 1999 position statement *Making decisions* the government indicated that it had no intention to legislate on advance directives at that time since "the guidance contained in case law, together with the Code of Practice, *Advance statements about medical treatment* (published by the BMA) provides sufficient clarity and flexibility to enable the validity and applicability of advance statements to be decided on a case by case basis".[32] The draft Mental Incapacity Bill it published in 2003, however, does contain provision to put advance refusals of treatment on a statutory footing. Information about any changes will be put on the BMA website (http://www.bma.org.uk/ethics).

12.6 Confidentiality

All patients have rights to privacy and to control information about themselves. In the case of people with impaired capacity, the principle of confidentiality must be balanced with protection of their interests.

Patients lacking capacity do not forfeit the right to control disclosure of personal information. They can authorise or prohibit the sharing of information about themselves if they broadly understand the implication of so doing. On the other hand, confidentiality is never absolute and, as with all patients, health professionals may have to consider breaching confidentiality, even in the face of a direct refusal by the patient, if there is a likelihood of foreseeable harm to the patient or others resulting from their silence.

Individual decision making about uses and disclosures of information is always to be encouraged, but inevitably carers and other people close to people who lack capacity are involved in helping them to make decisions and, so far as they are permitted to do so in their daily care of an individual, in taking decisions on the person's behalf. Increasing provision of care in the community means that more people have responsibilities in the provision of support for individuals lacking capacity. Nevertheless, unnecessary or widespread disclosure of identifiable personal health information without the individual's valid consent is not an appropriate response.

Disclosure without consent should normally be restricted to the sharing of essential information with those who have a demonstrable need to know it in order to provide proper care and supervision of the individual[33] (see also section 2.2). In exceptional cases there may be justification for the disclosure of information to other people to whom the incapacitated person may represent a potential health hazard, having first informed the patient of the intention to disclose. An example might be of a mentally incapable HIV-infected person embarking upon an intimate relationship. There can be no justification, however, for routine disclosure of that person's HIV-status to people whose contact with him or her contains no element of risk of infection.

The General Medical Council advises in the following way:

> Problems may arise if you consider that a patient is incapable of giving consent to treatment because of immaturity, illness or mental incapacity. If such patients ask you not to disclose information to a third party, you should try to persuade them to allow an appropriate person to be involved in the consultation. If they refuse and you are convinced that it is essential in the patient's medical interests, you may disclose relevant information to an appropriate person or authority. In such cases, you must tell the patient before disclosing any information and where appropriate, seek and carefully consider

the views of an advocate or carer. You should document in the patient's record the steps you have taken to obtain consent and the reasons for deciding to disclose information.

If you believe a patient to be a victim of neglect or physical or sexual abuse, and unable to give or withhold consent to disclosure, you should give information promptly to an appropriate responsible person or statutory agency, where you believe that disclosure is in the patient's best interests. You should usually inform the patient that you intend to disclose the information before doing so ... If for any reason, you believe that disclosure of information is not in the best interests of an abused or neglected person, you must still be prepared to justify your decision.[34]

Further information and guidance on confidentiality and disclosure of health information is available from the BMA[35] and from the Department of Health.[36]

12.7 Access to records

Under the Data Protection Act 1998, people have a statutory right of access to their own health records, or may authorise a third party, such as a lawyer, to do so on their behalf. Guidance on access to health records by patients, and in particular on the legal duties of doctors as holders of health records, has been issued by the BMA.[37] Where a person is deemed incapable of managing his or her property and affairs, access to relevant health information can be given to a person appointed by the Court of Protection to manage those affairs (see section 4.2.1 on the Court of Protection). In addition to the statutory provisions, health professionals have always exercised a discretionary ability to disclose information in the record to relevant people if they consider it would clearly be in the interests of the person lacking capacity to do so.

References and notes

1 There are various sources of guidance on consent to medical treatment which are summarised in: British Medical Association. *Consent tool kit, 2nd ed*. London: BMA, 2003. See also: Department of Health. *Reference guide to consent for examination or treatment*. London: DH, 2001; and Welsh Assembly Government. *Reference guide for consent to examination or treatment*. Cardiff: Welsh Assembly Government, 2002.

2   Department of Health, Welsh Office. *Mental Health Act 1983 code of practice*. London: The Stationery Office, 1999. In June 2002, the government issued for consultation a draft Mental Health Bill to extend the provisions for compulsory treatment to patients living in the community. The Bill provides for the publication of a new code of practice when new mental health legislation is introduced.

3   R v Bournewood Community and Mental Health NHS Trust, ex parte L [1998] 3 All ER 289.

4   Ibid: 305e

5   Department of Health. *Draft Mental Health Bill*. London: The Stationery Office, 2002: Part 5.

6   Re C (Adult: Refusal of Medical Treatment) [1994] 1 All ER 819.

7   Re MB (Medical Treatment) [1997] 2 FLR 426.

8   Ibid: 431c.

9   Sidaway v Board of Governors of the Bethlem Royal Hospital and Maudsley Hospital [1985] AC 871.

10 Re T (Adult: Refusal of Treatment) [1992] 4 All ER 649.

11 Ibid: 664j.

12 Ibid: 661h.

13 R v Collins and Ashworth Hospital Authority ex parte Brady [2001] 58 BMLR 173: 191.

14 Re F (Mental Patient: Sterilisation) [1990] 2 AC 1: 75H.

15 Ibid: 76G.

16 Re S (Sterilisation: Patient's Best Interests) [2000] 2 FLR 389.

17 Airedale NHS Trust v Bland [1993] AC 789.

18 Re F (Mental Patient: Sterilisation) [1990] 2 AC 1.

19 Re Y (Mental Incapacity: Bone Marrow Transplant) [1996] 2 FLR 787.

20 Re GF (Medical Treatment) [1992] 1 FLR 293.

21 Re SG (Adult Mental Patient: Abortion) [1991] 2 FLR 329. There may, however, be circumstances in which court involvement in a termination of pregnancy may be desirable. See for example: Re Doncaster and South Humberside Healthcare NHS Trust (2002) (unreported).

22 St George's Health Care NHS Trust v S, R v Collins and others, ex parte S [1998] 3 All ER 673: 703–704.

23 Re T (Adult: Refusal of Treatment) [1992] Op cit.

24 W v UK (1987) 10 EHRR 29.

25 British Medical Association. *Withholding and withdrawing life-prolonging medical treatment, 2nd ed*. London: BMJ Books, 2001.

26 Law Commission. *Mental incapacity*. London: HMSO, 1995. (Law Com No 231)

27 British Medical Association. *Advance statements about medical treatment*. London: BMA, 1995.

28 The Patients Association. *Living wills: a guide for patients*. London: Patients Association, 2003.

29 Airedale NHS Trust v Bland [1993]. Op cit. Re C (Adult: Refusal of Medical Treatment) [1994]. Op cit. Re T (Adult: Refusal of Treatment) [1992] Op cit.

30 Re T (Adult: Refusal of Treatment) [1992]. Op cit.

31 British Medical Association. *Advance statements about medical treatment*. Op cit.

32 Lord Chancellor's Department. *Making decisions: the government's proposals for making decisions on behalf of mentally incapacitated adults*. London: The Stationery Office, 1999: paragraph 20 (Cm 4465).

33 R (on the application of S) v Plymouth City Council [2002] 1 WLR 2583.

34 General Medical Council. *Confidentiality: protecting and providing information.* London: GMC, 2000: paras 38–39.
35 British Medical Association. *Confidentiality and disclosure of health information.* London: BMA, 1999.
36 Department of Health. *Confidentiality: NHS Code of Practice.* London: DH, 2003.
37 British Medical Association. *Access to health records by patients.* London: BMA, 2002.

13 Capacity to consent to research and innovative treatment

13.1 Introduction

A person's capacity to consent to research is assessed in the same way as capacity to consent to medical treatment (see Chapter 12). Additional safeguards, however, come into play, especially if the research involves any element of risk. This chapter considers the capacity of adults to agree to participate in research and the safeguards required for the involvement of adults who lack capacity to consent.

All research projects must be subject to the approval of an appropriate research ethics committee. Research also overlaps with the development of new or unproven medical or pharmaceutical interventions. New and innovative treatments often involve elements of both research and audit, so that their effectiveness and any risks or possible side effects can be properly assessed. Since 1998, the National Institute for Clinical Excellence (NICE) has also had a role in assessing the effectiveness of some treatments and therapies, both existing and innovative. In all projects involving research or innovative treatment, the safeguards to be applied must be commensurate with the risks involved.

13.2 Research governance

Traditionally, good practice in research and innovative treatment has been largely defined by guidance rather than law. Since the 1960s, following the World Medical Association's original Declaration of Helsinki[1] there has been a tendency to divide research procedures into two categories, the distinction being based on the intention of the researcher.

- First, procedures primarily aimed to benefit a particular patient but which incidentally also broadened knowledge of the condition or its treatment were classified as "therapeutic" research.

- Second, where the principal intention was to extend knowledge to benefit future patients but made no claim to benefit individual patients, the research was termed "non-therapeutic".

Accompanying the division into therapeutic and non-therapeutic research were strong reservations about allowing "vulnerable" patients, such as children or mentally incapacitated adults, to take part in research projects not intended to benefit them directly, while there was greater tolerance of their participation in so-called therapeutic research.

By 2000 it was increasingly argued that this categorisation was outmoded and misleading and should be dropped. For example, research guidance drawn up by the Royal College of Psychiatrists considered that such terms were not only unhelpful but that they also "disguised the fact that therapeutic research (for example a trial of a new drug) may often be considerably more hazardous than non-therapeutic research".[2] There was also concern that vulnerable patients were being excluded from research on their particular conditions and the benefits to be gained from it. In 2000, the World Medical Association deleted the terms from its guidance and set out general standards for all research to be assessed according to the same criteria of risks and benefits. The revised guidance also insisted that extra care and safeguards should be required when any research was combined with the care of patients.

In 2001 the way in which research (but not yet innovative treatment) was regulated began to change when the European Parliament approved a Directive to implement uniform rules on clinical trials of medicinal products and to require member states to harmonise their legislation to do this.[3] At the time of writing, the draft UK regulations had not been finalised, but the main proposals include the following:

- *good clinical practice* guidance must be observed[4]
- the foreseeable risks and inconveniences of a clinical trial must be weighed against the anticipated benefit for each subject in the trial and other present and future patients
- there must be provision for indemnity

- the rights of each subject to physical and mental integrity, privacy and protection of personal data must be safeguarded
- provision must be made for involvement of individuals who cannot consent
- a new statutory system for establishing and recognising research ethics committees should be established.[5]

Once implemented, more detailed information about the regulations will be available on the BMA website (http://www.bma.org.uk/ethics).

13.3 Capacity to consent to research

Consent is a key concept in research and innovative treatment. Whether or not individuals are able to give valid consent or refusal to a particular intervention depends upon the person's level of understanding and upon the provision of appropriate information about the procedure. The degree of detail required varies according to the needs of the individual patient and the complexity of the procedures involved. In particular, assessment of risk (an important part of decision making in all forms of health care) takes on greater significance in this sphere, since research and innovative treatment often involve a degree of uncertainty as to the risks involved. Ultimately, it is for the patient to decide whether to take the risk and participate in the research, having been given the fullest possible information. Individuals lack capacity to make a valid decision if:

- either they are unable to comprehend and retain the information which is material to the decision, especially as to the likely consequences of having or not having the procedure in question
- or they are unable to use the information and weigh it in the balance as part of the process of arriving at a decision.[6]

13.4 Research involving incompetent adults

Ideally, all research subjects should give well informed and considered consent to participation but, in practice, research cannot be limited to people who are able to decide for themselves, since the effect would be to deprive people who lack capacity of proven therapies for the conditions which specifically affect them. Many people with mental disorder are able to consent to research or innovative treatment if care is taken in explaining the procedures and risks involved. Nevertheless, the potential for exercising undue pressure or persuasion needs to be borne in mind, particularly where patients are detained in hospital or other institutions.

As a general principle, people who lack capacity to consent for themselves should only ever be involved in projects likely to benefit them directly or to benefit people in the same category and which cannot be undertaken on those who are able to consent. In such cases, research which is not contrary to the interests of the incapacitated person, which exposes them to no or only minimal risk, may not be unethical (see section 13.4.1 for the legal position) but must be subject to careful scrutiny by an appropriately constituted research ethics committee.

13.4.1 The legal position

Where adults lack capacity to consent in a valid way to participation in research, the legal position has long been that no other person is authorised to give proxy consent on their behalf (see section 12.4.4). Nevertheless (as discussed further below) the need to implement the European Directive on medicinal products meant that the UK had to make legal provision for a system of proxy consent. Although any such system of proxy consent under the Directive would only strictly apply to research on medicines (as opposed to research involving other forms of therapy, such as resuscitation techniques, or innovative surgery) in practice it seems likely that once proxy decision makers have been appointed they will be involved in other kinds of research decisions on behalf of incapacitated adults. Furthermore, it has long been accepted that research involving people who lack capacity is lawful where that participation is in their "best interests" (see section 12.4.2). In determining best interests, it is essential to consider the individual's previously expressed views whenever possible and, if feasible, that person's current wishes. Like the proxy decision making system, this often involves consulting relatives or other people emotionally close to the patient to try and discover the incapacitated individual's likely preferences.

Although the involvement of people lacking capacity in research not intended to benefit them directly has generally been regarded as ethical, provided certain safeguards are applied and the involvement is not contrary to the individual's interests, there continues to be doubt about its lawfulness. In 1995 the Law Commission concluded:

> If, however, the participant lacks capacity to consent to his or her participation, and the procedure cannot be justified under the doctrine of necessity, then any person who touches or restrains that participant is committing an unlawful battery. The simple fact is that the researcher is making no claim to be acting in the best interests of that individual person and does not therefore come within the rules of law set out in *Re F*.[7]

This issue has not been tested in court. As with other research or innovation, the research ethics committee must weigh carefully the expected benefits (such as early access to new therapies, increased nursing and medical attention, more frequent and regular health checks) against any potential risks and drawbacks.

As mentioned above, the European Directive on Clinical Trials has required the legal position to be clarified at least in relation to clinical trials of medicinal or pharmaceutical products. It states that:

> Persons who are incapable of giving legal consent to clinical trials should be given special protection. It is incumbent on the Member States to lay down rules to this effect. Such persons may not be included in clinical trials if the same results can be obtained using persons capable of giving consent ... In the case of other persons incapable of giving their consent, such as persons with dementia, psychiatric patients etc., inclusion in clinical trials should be on an even more restrictive basis. Medicinal products for trial may be administered to all such individuals only when there are grounds for assuming that the direct benefit to the patient outweighs the risks. Moreover in such cases the written consent of the patient's legal representative, given in cooperation with the treating doctor, is necessary before participation in any such clinical trial.[8]

Article 5 of the European Directive requires that the inclusion in clinical trials of incapacitated adults shall be allowed only if "the informed consent of a legal representative has been obtained".[9] In this context, a "legal representative" is someone with legal authority to act and not necessarily a lawyer. In the 2003 draft regulations intended to implement the European Directive in the UK, the government proposed a formal system of proxy decision making for incapacitated adults on the following lines.

- The provisions apply only to clinical trials of medicinal products and not to other forms of research or experimental therapy.
- The clinician in charge of the patient's care must believe the intervention to be in that person's best interests.
- Any advance refusal of treatment made by the person prior to the onset of incapacity must be respected.
- In the absence of such evidence it is suggested that consent to interventions deemed to be in the patient's interests could be provided by a "legal representative". Two types of representative are envisaged:

  - "personal" representatives who have a relationship with the patient
  - "professional" representatives who can act if there is no suitable person to act as a personal representative.[10]

The government has promised to provide guidance for "legal representatives" when the regulations come into effect and, when available, such information will be reflected in the advice published on the BMA website (http://www.bma.org.uk/ethics).

13.5 Innovative treatment

Innovative treatments are often an extension of usual treatments but they may expose the patient to a greater degree of risk than established procedures. An experienced surgeon, for example, may modify a particular surgical procedure for an individual patient if a superior outcome might be expected from the modification. Efforts should be made to inform patients, so far as they are able to understand, how and why the proposed treatment differs from the usual measures and the known or likely risks attached. They should also be given any relevant information about the success rate of the treating clinician.

Innovative treatments are usually a standard feature of medical practice and the fact that useful information is gained as a by-product is seen as largely incidental. Nevertheless, participation of incapacitated people in new treatments whose risks they may not be able to fully appreciate obviously needs to be carefully monitored. Indeed, involving incapacitated patients in innovative therapies which have not previously been tested on fully consenting adults or where there are likely to be significant risks gives rise to legal and ethical uncertainty. It is recommended that in any instance where a doctor proposes a procedure which diverges substantially from accepted practice, involving an unknown or increased risk, advance expert scrutiny of the ethics and legality of the procedure should be carried out. In some circumstances, a court declaration may be required.

The search for effective treatment of Creutzfeldt–Jakob disease (CJD) provides an example of the type of situation where court intervention may be required. In December 2002 a court was asked to decide whether it would be lawful to provide treatment that had not been tested on human beings to two young patients who were thought to be suffering from variant CJD. Both patients (JS aged 18 and JA aged 16) lacked the capacity to make treatment decisions, but their parents argued that it would be in their best interests to have the new therapy. The treatment had been tested in a Japanese research project but only on animals, but was soon to be given to Japanese patients with iatrogenic CJD. Although not expected to provide a cure, it was hoped that the treatment could improve patients' lives. The judge said that although the patients would not recover, the concept of "benefit" to a patient suffering from variant CJD would encompass any of the following:

- an improvement from the present state of illness
- a continuation of the existing state of illness without deterioration for a longer period than might otherwise have occurred
- the prolongation of life for a longer period than might otherwise have occurred.

Given the possibility of some benefit being derived and the lack of any other alternative, it was held that this treatment would be in the best interests of both JS and JA and so could lawfully be provided.[11]

13.6 Proposals for law reform

The Law Commission has recommended that the legal position concerning the involvement of vulnerable adults in research projects should be clarified. It proposed that research which is unlikely to benefit a participant, or whose benefit is likely to be long delayed, should be lawful if (a) the research is into an incapacitating condition with which the person is or may be affected, and (b) certain statutory procedures are complied with. The statutory procedures referred to relate primarily to obtaining the approval of a new statutory committee.[12] Nevertheless, in its policy statement *Making decisions* published in 1999[13] and in the subsequent draft Mental Incapacity Bill published in 2003 there were no proposals to include any such provisions to change the law with regard to medical research. No reason was given for this omission.

Although the European Clinical Trials Directive has required the government to harmonise UK legislation governing the clinical trials of medicinal products with that in force in other EU member states (see section 13.4.1) the legal position regarding the participation of incapacitated adults in other areas of research and innovative treatment remains uncertain at the time of writing.

References and notes

1 World Medical Association. *Declaration of Helsinki.* Ferney-Voltaire: WMA, 1964 (and subsequent amendments).
2 Royal College of Psychiatrists. *Guidelines for researchers and ethics committees on psychiatric research involving human participants.* London: RCPsych, 2000: 8.
3 Directive 2001/20/EC of the European Parliament and of the Council of 4 April 2001 on the approximation of the laws, regulations and administrative provisions of the member states relating to the implementation of good clinical practice in the conduct of clinical trials on medicinal products for human use. *Official Journal of the European Communities* 2001;L121: 34–44.

4   European Agency for the Evaluation of Medicinal Products. *Note for guidance on good clinical practice (CPMP/ICH/95)*. London: EMEA, 1996.
5   The Medicines for Human Use (Clinical Trials) Regulations 2003 (draft).
6   The test of capacity to consent to research or innovative treatment is the same as that involved in treatment decisions, as set out in: Re MB (Medical Treatment) [1997] 2 FLR 426.
7   Law Commission. *Mental incapacity*. London: HMSO, 1995: paragraph 6.29. (Law Com No 231) This was based on the "best interests" test set out in Re F (Mental Patient: Sterilisation) [1990] 2 AC 1.
8   Directive 2001/20/EC of the European Parliament and of the Council of 4 April 2001 on the approximation of the laws, regulations and administrative provisions of the member states relating to the implementation of good clinical practice in the conduct of clinical trials on medicinal products for human use. Op cit: preamble, paragraphs 3 and 4.
9   Ibid: Article 5(a).
10 Medicines for Human Use (Clinical Trials) Regulations 2003 (draft).
11 Simms v Simms, PA v JA (Also known as: A v A, JS v An NHS Trust) [2003] 1 All ER 669.
12 Law Commission. *Mental incapacity*. Op cit: Part VI.
13 Lord Chancellor's Department. *Making decisions: the government's proposals for making decisions on behalf of mentally incapacitated adults*. London: The Stationery Office, 1999: paragraph 12 (Cm 4465).

Part IV
Practical aspects of the assessment of capacity

Part IV deals with the medical practicalities of assessing capacity. Chapter 14 sets out accepted practice for carrying out assessments of capacity and will be familiar to medical practitioners who regularly work in the mental health field. It is primarily intended to assist health professionals who only occasionally encounter a request for an assessment of capacity to be carried out. Chapter 15 aims to help lawyers direct their requests for a medical opinion appropriately and to be aware of the steps involved in a medical assessment.

Accurate assessment depends upon clarity on the part of both lawyers and doctors about the relationship between legal and medical concepts. It therefore depends upon doctors knowing something about the law and lawyers understanding something of medical assessment and diagnosis. Both chapters in Part IV should therefore be read as two sides of a single coin.

14 Practical guidelines for doctors

14.1 Introduction

Doctors have great powers to benefit their patients by providing them with effective treatments. Doctors may also be able to help protect patients from exploitation and abuse by identifying medical conditions which may affect their ability to protect themselves. They also risk doing harm to patients, however, if their treatments are unsuccessful, or if their diagnoses or actions result in depriving patients of the right to make their own decisions. In all their work doctors have to balance the risks of doing damage against the possible advantages of intervention, and similar dilemmas arise in the assessment of capacity. Although guidance is available and new clinical assessment tools are being developed (particularly in the USA[1]), their application is not always clear-cut and there is a need for careful consideration in every case.

Capacity is a legal concept and the tests which are applied to determine whether a person has any particular capacity originate in law. Ultimately, the decision about a person's capacity can be decided by a court. In practice, however, doctors frequently give opinions about capacity which are accepted without further legal intervention. A doctor may be required:

- to make an assessment of a patient's capacity to consent prior to giving or prescribing medical treatment
- to provide a medical certificate or opinion, at a solicitor's request, as to a particular capacity unrelated to medical treatment
- to witness or otherwise certify a legal document signed by someone
- to give an opinion as to a particular capacity which is relevant to other legal proceedings.

Doctors are also frequently asked to advise about other capacities for which there are no specific legal tests. One matter on which doctors' opinions are frequently sought is whether an infirm elderly person is able to continue to live in his or her own home or whether a move to sheltered housing or a care home is advisable. The doctor's assessment in such cases would cover the person's physical and mental abilities relating to personal care and welfare as well as his or her capacity to make the decision, and should be based on information provided by the individual concerned, family members and carers as well as other relevant factors. Refusal to leave his or her own home, even when this is considered by others to be contrary to the person's best interests, is not in itself evidence of incapacity and the decision should be respected, unless lack of capacity is otherwise demonstrated. In certain limited circumstances, there may be grounds for compulsory admission to hospital or nursing care under mental health legislation.

Irrespective of whether doctors are assessing the capacity to consent to medical treatment or a capacity which is in a different area unrelated to medical treatment, they should make careful reference to the relevant legal criteria (see Part III). Where assessments are carried out at the request of a solicitor or other legal professional, doctors should insist that the lawyer is explicit about the particular question which is to be answered. They must also ensure that any legal jargon is properly explained by the lawyer and that they are given all necessary information to be able to complete the assessment. For example if a doctor is asked to assess a person's capacity to make a will, he or she needs details of the extent of the person's assets and members of the person's family and any other people who may have a claim on the testator's estate (see Chapter 5).

Doctors should then assess whether the person's mental capacity is adequate to satisfy the relevant legal criteria. It is important for doctors to recognise that there may also be non-medical evidence about a person's capacity, which may sometimes contradict their own medical view. This emphasises that the doctor's role is to give an opinion – rather than to be the sole arbiter as to capacity.[2] Any medical opinion about capacity is open to legal challenge, either by the person whose capacity is being assessed, or by some other interested party, and – ultimately – the doctor can be called to give evidence in court. Doctors are therefore advised to keep careful records of the steps taken in assessing capacity.

14.2 Defining capacity

Capacity is the ability to do something. In a legal context it refers to a person's ability to do something, including making a decision, which may have legal consequences for the person him or herself or for other people (see Chapter 1). Capacity is the pivotal issue in balancing the right to autonomy in decision making and the right to protection from harm.

An assessment of capacity is not based upon the test "would a rational person decide as this person has decided?". It is not the decision itself but the thought processes which lie behind the decision which are relevant to the question of capacity. Individuals who have mental capacity may make decisions which are apparently irrational and the law allows them to do so. There is a presumption that a person has capacity until the contrary is proven and also that a person who has been shown to lack a legal capacity is generally assumed to remain incapable until the contrary is proven (see section 3.2.1). Since the "presumption of capacity" must be the starting point of any assessment, lack of cooperation or apathy with respect to an assessment of capacity should not lead to a conclusion that the person lacks capacity. For example, an eccentric recluse does not lose legal autonomy simply because of non-cooperation with an assessment (see section 2.4 on refusal to be assessed).

Existing legal tests of capacity do not necessarily look to whether there is a diagnosable medical condition. What is important is the ability of the person to pass the relevant test (see Part III for existing legal tests). Where there is a medical disorder, it is not a diagnosis which implies capacity or incapacity but, rather, the person's specific disabilities. Similarly, different legal capacities can be variously affected by a particular medical disability. For example a diagnosis of schizophrenia does not determine whether or not a person lacks a particular capacity. A person with schizophrenia may have the capacity to accept or refuse some medical treatments but not others, depending upon the nature of his or her symptoms.[3] More generally, a person may have the capacity to carry out one type of legal act, such as marrying, whilst not having the capacity to carry out another, such as making a will.[4]

A person's capacity is largely determined by that person's mental state. There may also be some physical condition, such as severe pain or fatigue, which does not directly affect mental functioning but which can sometimes interfere with capacity. Poor eyesight, deafness and problems with speech and language may be relevant to whether a person's wishes can be ascertained. Every effort must be made to overcome such problems with perception and communication.

The Law Commission has recommended that its test of capacity should require that a person's inability to make a decision is linked to the presence of a "mental disability", except in cases where the person is unable to communicate.[5] The arguments for and against such a diagnostic hurdle are very finely balanced and they are set out in full in the Law Commission's Consultation Paper No. 128.[6] There appears to be good reason to agree with the Law Commission's view that a diagnostic hurdle does have a role to play in any definition of incapacity, in particular in ensuring that the test is stringent enough not to catch large numbers of people who make unusual or unwise decisions.

Where it is not clear that a person has capacity to make a decision, doctors have to balance the need to protect the person from harm against the possibility of doing good; whatever assessment they make could be criticised or challenged and should therefore be carefully documented and their findings recorded.

14.3 The doctor's role

Although assessing any particular capacity does not require detailed legal knowledge, the doctor must understand in broad terms the relevant legal tests. The doctor's role is to supply information on which an assessment of the person's legal capacity can be based. The doctor needs to describe the consequences of medical conditions which may compromise an individual's ability to pass a legal test. If there is no medical diagnosis there can be no relevant medical evidence as to capacity. For example, to say that a person "makes poor judgments" is not a medical opinion, but a lay observation, and one which is heavily subjective. This emphasises the importance of the doctor first of all determining that it is appropriate to give a medical opinion about capacity.

Although a doctor may be asked to give an opinion about capacity, this opinion is not necessarily the deciding factor – evidence from other people and other sources also needs to be taken into account. Also, some tests of capacity make explicit or implicit reference to social functioning rather than to medical disabilities per se (see for example Chapter 10 on personal relationships) and a doctor is no more expert at assessing social functioning than anyone else.

Where the relevant legal capacity is the capacity to consent to specific medical treatment, doctors should take particular care and have regard to the professional and other guidance available (see also Chapter 12).[7] The doctor may be in a situation where his or her opinion of the patient's best interests conflicts with what the patient wants. It is tempting, but ethically and legally wrong, for the doctor to underestimate the capacity of the patient in order to achieve what the doctor believes to be in that person's best interests. In so doing, the doctor deprives the patient of his or her autonomy.

14.3.1 Professional ethics

There are two distinct contexts in which doctors examine people. The most common is the therapeutic context to ensure that patients receive appropriate care and treatment. Patient consent is normally implicit, as is permission to disclose to other health professionals such information as is essential for the provision of care. Nevertheless, patients must be informed about the scope of disclosure within the therapeutic context, since care is increasingly provided by multi-disciplinary teams and information may be spread more widely than patients anticipate (see sections 2.2 and 12.6 on confidentiality).

The second situation is where doctors act as independent examiners in order to provide a report for purposes other than treatment, for example for use in legal proceedings. When a doctor is carrying out this second type of assessment, patient consent to examination and to disclosure of information cannot be assumed. It is essential that the doctor's role and the purpose of the exercise are explained to the person at the outset. No-one can legally consent to examination on behalf of an adult, but relatives may help ensure that the person understands the situation.

Ensuring clarity is particularly difficult when assessment for a report to third parties is carried out by the patient's own doctor and takes place within the context of a continuing therapeutic relationship. In such cases, the doctor must explain how the examination differs from the usual doctor–patient encounter and obtain explicit patient consent. Patients must also be told who will have access to the information gained and whether other material from their past records will be needed. The patient's consent to such disclosure should be recorded.

If an individual appears competent and refuses to cooperate with assessment, the doctor must note that fact in conjunction with the other evidence available (see also section 2.4). If it appears likely that the person lacks capacity to consent to assessment or to disclosure, the doctor should take a decision whether or not to proceed with the assessment based on a judgment of the person's best interests. Such judgment necessarily includes appropriate weight being given to the ascertainable past and current wishes of that individual.

14.3.2 Which doctor should assess the person?

In a joint report aimed at tackling stigmatisation and discrimination in the medical profession against people with mental health problems, the BMA, the Royal College of Physicians and the Royal College of Psychiatrists have called for organisations with responsibility for training and accreditation to develop clear guidance for all doctors concerning the need to acquire knowledge and skills related to the recognition and management of mental illness, comparable to those required in respect of all other illnesses.[8] They also propose that medical education and training, including continuing professional development, should ensure that all doctors have the relevant competencies (in terms of attitude, skills and knowledge) for examining an individual's mental state, comparable to competence in examining physical state. Doctors should only give an opinion of a person's mental capacity where they feel competent to do so.

The choice of doctor to make an assessment of capacity depends on the particular requirements of the assessment and the medical condition of the person being assessed. Many people can be assessed by their general practitioner, and indeed in some cases, a close, long-term acquaintance with the person being assessed may be an asset, particularly if that person is more relaxed with a familiar doctor. On some occasions, however, the GP's personal knowledge of a patient, and perhaps also of the patient's family, may make an objective assessment more difficult. If the nature or complexity of the person's medical disorder or disabilities suggests that a hospital specialist would be more appropriate then it is usually important for that doctor to obtain information from the person's GP, and take this into account in making his or her own assessment of the patient's capacity. Other members of the multi-disciplinary team, particularly nurses, clinical psychologists and occupational therapists may also have specific skills to assist the doctor in assessing capacity.

Whoever carries out the assessment should make efforts to create the most congenial environment, to optimise the conditions for assessing the person's capacity at their highest level of functioning (see sections 2.3 and 14.7).

14.4 A systematic approach to assessing capacity

14.4.1 Background information

Once sure of the relevant legal test, the assessing doctor should become familiar with any background information about the person likely to be relevant to that particular test. The amount of information required is determined by the complexity of the legal decision to be taken. For example, if the assessment relates to the capacity to make a will, the assessing doctor needs to have some idea about the extent and complexity of the person's estate and whether the person understands the claims of others to which consideration should be given in deciding about disposal of his or her assets (see Chapter 5). The doctor must therefore have some knowledge of the number and nature of claims on the individual. Although the medical assessment should be carried out with an eye to the relevant legal criteria, there must be a clear distinction between the description of the disabilities and the interpretation of how they affect legal capacity. The doctor should, therefore, first define the diagnosis and the medical disabilities and then assess how these affect the person's ability to pass the relevant legal test of capacity.

14.4.2 Medical records and reports

Prior to undertaking an assessment, the doctor should try to have access to all relevant past medical and psychiatric records. An understanding of the progression of the person's disease is relevant to prognosis, to any likely response to treatment, and thus to future potential capacity. Assessment of the permanence or transience of disabilities may be crucially important in offering a view about achievable capacity. Also, the medical records may give a different picture of a person's disabilities in general terms from the impression the doctor gains at an individual assessment. It is important, however, for the doctor to make an assessment on the basis of current evidence from various information sources, rather than relying entirely on past evaluations.

The doctor should also take full account of relevant information from other disciplines. An assessment by a clinical psychologist may already be available, or could be sought, and this may assist in giving a detailed, validated and systematic assessment of cognitive functioning. An occupational therapist might be consulted when information about activities of daily living is of importance. Also, a report from a social worker, a nurse or a care worker may be helpful, for example where the person is living in a care home.

14.4.3 Information from others

Information from friends, relatives or carers is often of great importance in the assessment of disability and its progression. Great care must be taken, however, when gaining information from such third parties, particularly if they have an interest in the outcome of the assessment of capacity. It is also important to take account of the person's known previous patterns of behaviour, values, and goals. These may give clues as to whether current behaviour and thinking reflects an abnormal mental state. Aspects of a person's current thinking may derive not from a medical disability but from a normal personality, or from a particular cultural or ethnic background, and this may be of importance in determining capacity. It may even be necessary for the doctor to seek advice from others on such cultural issues, or to suggest that the patient be examined by a doctor of a cultural or ethnic background similar to the person being assessed.[9]

14.4.4 Medical diagnosis

Where the person suffers from a mental disorder, it is good practice to express the diagnosis in terms of one of the accepted international classifications of mental disorders, the World Health Organization's international classification of diseases (WHO ICD-10), or the American Psychiatric Association's diagnostic and statistical manual (DSM-IV). This will ensure greater diagnostic consistency between doctors and minimise diagnostic confusion.

14.5 The mental state in relation to capacity

Examination of the mental state is fundamental to the assessment of capacity. Although particular diagnoses may tend to be associated with particular mental state disabilities which affect capacity, what matters are the disabilities themselves. It is only through detailed assessment of specific aspects of mental functioning that capacity can be properly assessed.

14.5.1 Mental state examination

The doctor should consider the patient's mental functioning under the following headings when making an assessment of the mental state, indicating the relevance of any findings to the specific test of capacity. It is also important to document any medical or psychometric tests or other assessment tools used in the process.[10]

Appearance and behaviour

A patient may be so agitated or overactive in his or her behaviour that it may be impossible to impart relevant information. Otherwise, appearance and behaviour may suggest a mood disorder or cognitive impairment which might be relevant to the person's capacity.

Speech

The rate, quantity, form or flow of speech may be such as to interfere with communication, as well as reflecting abnormality of thought processes. For example, a depressed patient may be so lacking in speech as to be unable to communicate effectively; or a manic patient's speech may be rapid with quickly changing subjects ("flight of ideas") so that communication is severely impaired. Similarly, the thought disorder of a schizophrenic patient (moving between topics without apparent logical connections) may make communication very difficult or even impossible. Damage to the language areas of the brain following a stroke may also make direct verbal communication impossible.

Mood

Mood may be very important in determining capacity. A depressed patient with delusions of poverty may make decisions relevant to his or her affairs on an entirely erroneous basis. Similarly, the grandiose approach of a hypomanic patient may lead to rash financial or other decisions. Lability of mood (common after a stroke) may render a patient unable to make consistent decisions. Anxiety may also have some effect on the assessed level of capacity.

Thought

Abnormalities of thought may have a profound effect upon decision making. Delusions which are strongly held, and which relate specifically to the decision at hand, may substantially distort a person's ability to make the decision. For example, someone's capacity to make a will might be affected by a delusional belief that a close relative is plotting against him or her. Similarly, a delusional belief that doctors have magical powers to cure may render a patient incapable of consenting to medical treatment. Thought abnormalities falling short of delusions (for example, extreme preoccupation or obsessional thoughts) can also interfere with capacity but are less likely to do so. Overvalued ideas falling short of delusions (such as occur in anorexia nervosa) present particular difficulties in relation to the capacity of such patients to consent to treatment or to accept or refuse food.

Perception

Illusions (misinterpretation of the nature of real objects) are rarely significant enough to inhibit capacity. Hallucinations, however, may well be of direct relevance to decision making. They are often congruent with, or reinforce, delusions and so the two should be considered together. Auditory hallucinations instructing the patient may have two distinct effects. Firstly, by their content and authority they may directly interfere with the patient's ability to think about relevant issues as well as with the decision making ability. Secondly, hallucinations may be so incessant that they distract the person from thinking about the decision at all.

Cognition

Defects in cognitive functioning can have profound significance for capacity. Decision making and all tests of legal capacity require not only consciousness but some continuity of consciousness and of recollection. Attention (the ability to focus on the matter in hand) and concentration (the ability to sustain attention) are necessary for effective thought and for capacity. Patients who are highly distracted, whether by other mental events such as hallucinations or because of delirium, may lack capacity. Most psychiatrists use the Mini-Mental State Examination (MMSE) as a convenient way of assessing different domains of cognitive function.[11] If this test reveals areas of impairment it may be helpful to make a more detailed appraisal of the affected cognitive abilities.

Orientation

Awareness of time, place and person, might be seen as relevant only to set the context for decisions rather than being directly relevant to capacity. Disorientation, however, is usually a marker of brain dysfunction, for instance in delirium or dementia, and in these conditions capacity is commonly impaired.

Memory

Problems with long-term memory may not necessarily reduce capacity. A person who cannot remember his or her relatives or the extent of financial assets, however, could be significantly impaired in decision making ability. A person with a severe short-term memory deficit (an inability to recall information given a few minutes earlier) which may occur as a result of chronic alcoholism, a stroke, or Alzheimer's disease, is likely to lack capacity for some – but not necessarily all – decisions.

Intelligence

Limited intelligence (for example as a result of learning disability) may reduce capacity for certain decisions, although it may be possible to use aids to communication, such as pictures or videos to enhance understanding. Care should be taken not to presume incapacity just because the person has a learning disability. There should be careful investigation of the person's abilities specifically in relation to the decision in question. Acquired brain damage, whether from trauma or from disease processes affecting the brain, may also affect cognitive functioning and, therefore, capacity. Where, however, only certain aspects of intellectual functioning are significantly impaired it is important to be very specific in distinguishing which functions, or combination of functions, are necessary for the legal capacity which the person must have. Standardised psychometric tests may be of help in assessing the severity of cognitive impairment. Many simple tests of cognitive functioning assess only orientation and memory, but it is important also to assess other areas of mental functioning, such as calculation, reasoning, visuospatial functioning, and sequencing. An occupational therapist or clinical psychologist may be able to help in these areas.

Insight

People can lack insight into one aspect of their lives and retain it for others. For example, lack of insight as to the presence of illness might not deprive a person of the capacity to make decisions about treatment of the illness if the person has insight into the need for such treatment. Furthermore, insight may not be completely absent. The person with reduced insight may have specific awareness of his or her condition so as to have the capacity necessary for decisions about treatment. Of course, lack of insight into mental illness may not inhibit the person's capacity to decide about something else in his or her life. No report should read "has insight" or "has no insight"; if unqualified, either statement is valueless.

14.6 Personality disorders

By contrast with mental illness or organic brain syndromes, personality disorders present particular problems in relation to assessment of capacity. Such patients have disorders which affect many areas of mental and social functioning, as well as behaviour. They often experience profound mood disturbances and are frequently impulsive. Their thought processes are unusual, but they are not deluded. It is the manner in which persons weigh decisions in the balance which is generally affected, not their ability to think.[12] Assessment of capacity in such patients is extremely difficult since there are no clear-cut abnormalities in the mental state, such as hallucinations or delusions, and yet the doctor often perceives that they are not making decisions in the way that an ordinary person would. There should be no automatic assumption that this necessarily indicates impaired capacity.

14.7 The duty to enhance mental capacity

Doctors are aware both that medical disabilities can fluctuate and that there are many factors other than a person's medical disorder which may adversely influence capacity. It is the duty of the assessing doctor to optimise the conditions to allow the person's capacity to be assessed at his or her highest level of functioning in relation to the decision in question.

Some pointers to assist in creating the best environment for assessing capacity are suggested in section 2.3. Further elaboration on the relevant pointers for doctors is set out here.

- Any treatable medical condition which affects capacity should as far as possible be treated before a final assessment is made.

- Incapacity may be temporary, albeit for a prolonged period. For example, an older patient with delirium caused by infection may continue to improve for some time after the infection has been eradicated. If a person's condition is likely to improve the assessment of capacity should, if possible, be delayed. The effect of drugs, particularly hypnotics and tranquillisers, should be considered carefully. If there is a treatable physical disorder present, assessment should be delayed until the patient is as well and comfortable as possible.

- Some conditions, such as dementia with Lewy bodies, may give rise to fluctuating capacity. Thus, although a person with dementia may lack capacity at the time of an assessment; the result may be different if a second assessment is undertaken during a lucid interval. In cases of fluctuating capacity the medical report should detail the level of capacity during periods of maximal and minimal disability.

- Some mental disabilities may be untreatable and yet their impact can be minimised. For example, the capacity of a person with a short-term memory deficit to make a particular decision may be improved if trained in suitable techniques by an occupational therapist or psychologist. If the assessing doctor believes that capacity could be improved by such assistance then this should be stated in any opinion.

- Some physical conditions which do not directly affect the mental state can appear to interfere with capacity. For example, disabilities of communication do not impair the ability to understand relevant information or make a choice, but they may prevent the person's wishes being made known. Many communication difficulties which result from physical disabilities can be helped. There should, therefore, be careful assessment of speech, language functioning, hearing and (if appropriate) sight. Any disabilities discovered should as far as possible (and if time allows) be corrected before any conclusion is reached about capacity.

- Care should be taken to choose the best location and time for the assessment. For someone who is on the borderline of having capacity, anxiety may tip that person into apparent incapacity. It may be appropriate to do the assessment in the person's own home if it is thought that an interview at either a hospital or a GP's surgery would adversely affect the result. A relative or carer may be able to indicate the most suitable location and time for the assessment.

- The way in which someone is approached and dealt with generally can have a significant impact upon apparent capacity and the doctor should be sensitive to this.
- Educating the person who is being assessed as to the factors relevant to the proposed decision may enhance capacity. Indeed, the assessing doctor should always establish what the person understands about the decision he or she is being asked to undertake. It is important for the doctor to re-explain and, if necessary, write down those aspects of the decision which have not been fully grasped. The person being assessed should be allowed sufficient time to become familiar with concepts relevant to the decision. For example, people with learning disabilities may acquire the capacity to consent to a blood test after receiving appropriate information in an accessible manner.[13]
- The capacity of some people may be enhanced by the presence of a friend, relative, or other person at the interview. Alternatively, the presence of a third party may increase the anxiety and thus reduce the person's capacity. The person being assessed should be asked specifically whether he or she would feel more comfortable with another person present. A professional advocate may be able to ensure that the person's views have been adequately represented.
- Depression is common amongst those with other disabilities but is often not recognised. Its presence may profoundly affect capacity and yet it may be amenable to treatment. Making a diagnosis of depression in the presence of other disabilities affecting mental functioning can be particularly difficult, especially in patients with dementia. The opinion of a psychiatrist may be necessary in such cases. The low self-esteem of many patients whose capacity may be in question means that they are at particular risk of "going along with" suggestions regardless of their own private views. The assessing doctor should be aware of this and structure the interview so as to avoid the use of leading questions.

14.8 Retrospective assessment

On occasions a doctor may be asked to advise whether a person had the capacity some time in the past to make a decision which he or she made. Examples might be the capacity to make a will (see Chapter 5) where the person subsequently dies, or capacity to enter into a contract (see Chapter 8) where the validity of the contract is subsequently challenged. Any such retrospective assessment has to be based upon medical notes made at the time, as well as on other non-medical information which may help to suggest the nature of the person's mental functioning at the time, and whether he or she may have been susceptible to the exertion of undue influence or pressure.

14.9 General guidance

Assessment of capacity is not a function which can usually be carried out in only a few minutes. Aside from situations where the patient is comatose, or otherwise so severely disabled that incapacity is obvious, assessment usually takes a substantial period of time, even if only a single area of capacity is to be explored. This is required both because of the need to be thorough and comprehensive and because of the legal importance which attaches to the assessment. The doctor should never be constrained in making assessment by time or resources. Each assessment of capacity must be an assessment of an individual in his or her own circumstances. No assumptions should be made about capacity just on the basis of the person's known diagnosis. What matters is how the medical condition affects the particular person's own capacity, not the diagnosed medical condition itself. It is worth emphasising again that the doctor must guard against allowing a personal view of what is in the person's best interests to influence an assessment of capacity. It may be disconcerting for the doctor to determine that the patient has capacity when the doctor believes that allowing the patient to make the decision will be against the patient's long-term interests. The doctor must not, however, consider the implications of the person being allowed to make the decision, except to the extent that this is relevant in deciding whether the person has the capacity to do so.

References and notes

1   The assessment tools being developed in the USA and their application in the UK are reviewed in: Eastman N, Dhar R. The role of assessment of mental capacity: a review. *Curr Opin Psychiatry* 2000;**13**:557–61.
2   Richmond v Richmond (1914) 111 LT 273.
3   Re C (Adult: Refusal of Medical Treatment) [1994] 1 All ER 819.
4   In the Estate of Park, Park v Park [1954] P 112.
5   Law Commission. *Mental incapacity*. London: HMSO, 1995: paragraph 3.12 (Law Com No 231).
6   Law Commission. *Mental incapacity: a new jurisdiction?* London: HMSO, 1993: paragraphs 3.7–3.14 (Law Com No 128).
7   There are various sources of guidance on consent to medical treatment which are summarised in: British Medical Association. *Consent tool kit, 2nd ed*. London: BMA, 2003. See also: Department of Health. *Reference guide to consent for examination or treatment*. London: DoH, 2001. And: Welsh Assembly Government. *Reference guide for consent to examination or treatment*. Cardiff: Welsh Assembly Government, 2002.
8   Royal College of Psychiatrists, Royal College of Physicians of London, British Medical Association. *Mental illness: stigmatisation and discrimination within the medical profession*. London: RCPsych, 2001 (Council Report CR91).
9   See for example: Fernando S, ed. *Mental health in a multi-ethnic society*. London: Routledge, 1995. And: Bashir Q. *Transcultural medicine: dealing with patients from different cultures, 2nd ed*. London: Kluwer Academic Publishers, 1994.
10 See for example: Folstein MF, Folstein SE, McHugh PR. "Mini-mental state": a practical method for grading the cognitive state of patients for the clinician. *J Psychiatr Res* 1975;**12**:189–98. Also: Grisso T, Appelbaum PS, Hill-Fotouhi C. The MacCAT-T: a clinical tool to assess patients' treatment decisions. *Psychiat Serv* 1997;**48**:1315–9. And: Janofsky JS, McCarthy RJ, Folstein MF. The Hopkins competency assessment test. *Hosp Community Psychiat* 1992;**43**:132–6.
11 Folstein MF, Folstein SE, McHugh PR. "Mini-mental state": a practical method for grading the cognitive state of patients for the clinician. Op cit.
12 It has been held that severe personality disorder alone could be sufficient to have "eschewed the weighing of information and the balancing of risks and needs to such an extent that ... his decisions on food refusal and force feeding had been incapacitated". R v Collins and Ashworth Hospital Authority ex parte Brady (2001) 58 BMLR 173: 191.
13 Wong JG, Clare ICH, Gunn MJ, Holland AJ. Capacity to make health care decisions: its importance in clinical practice. *Psychol Med* 1999;**29**: 437–46.

15 Practical guidelines for lawyers

15.1 Introduction

In cases where a client's mental capacity is in doubt, it is often desirable, or a matter of good practice, for lawyers to obtain a medical or other expert opinion. Indeed, in some circumstances obtaining medical evidence about a person's capacity is required by law (see section 3.5.1). Lawyers must be clear about which kind of doctor to ask to give an expert opinion about any particular legal capacity. They need to explain in detail which particular areas of capacity they wish the doctor to report on, as individuals may have some capacities but not others.[1] They should also clarify for the doctor the relevant legal tests of capacity as described in Part III. Where the particular test of capacity has been established in case law, it may sometimes be appropriate to send to the medical practitioner the actual text of the relevant judgment. In all cases, it is important that any summary of the law is understandable to someone who is not a lawyer, and in a form which would be acceptable to the courts. Unless such detailed information is given, doctors are likely to refer back to medical textbooks to find out what is required, and medical texts cannot be relied upon in a legal context. Appendix G is a sample letter of instruction for a medical report which can be adapted depending on the test of capacity required. Copies of articles or extracts of law reports can be attached and referred to in the letter of instruction, and may assist the doctor in the preparation of a helpful and relevant assessment.

It is also necessary to describe the client's circumstances where these are relevant to the person's capacity to make the decision in question. For example, if testamentary capacity is to be assessed it is necessary for the doctor to be given some independent information about the extent of the testator's assets, and those who may have a call on the estate, and perhaps a draft of the proposed will (see Chapter 5). This is particularly relevant where the doctor is asked to witness the will in accordance with the so-called "golden rule" (see sections 3.5.1 and 5.4). In any situation where doctors or nurses are asked to witness documents, it is important to emphasise to them that they are expected to use their professional skills in attesting the patient's competence to sign, and not merely acting as lay witnesses (see section 3.5).

It is often helpful for there to be a discussion between lawyer and doctor prior to the doctor's consideration of the case, both to clarify the legal questions and to establish what documentary information is available which the doctor should see. It is also helpful for lawyers to have some knowledge of the basic principles which underlie medical assessment in order both to evaluate the opinion and to be sure of understanding its legal implications. A summary is set out in section 15.4 and further details are given in Chapter 14.

As a matter of good practice, lawyers who visit clients in hospitals or care homes or doctors who visit to carry out an assessment should notify the ward or home in advance of their expected visit and introduce themselves to the duty manager to ascertain that the client is well enough to receive a professional visit. While clients' access to their legal advisers should not be hindered, lawyers need to be sensitive to the client's condition and medical needs and arrange an appropriate time to visit.

The remainder of this chapter offers basic information about different specialities and medical personnel, and about the nature of psychiatric assessment and diagnosis.

15.2 Who should assess the person?

The only grounds on which a doctor can offer an expert opinion is when the person being assessed suffers (or appears to suffer) from a diagnosable medical condition. Lawyers should therefore be wary of any assessment which appears to be "medical" but which has nothing to do with medical disabilities.

Mental disabilities can arise from either "physical" or "psychiatric" conditions. Any doctor should be able to take a psychiatric history and to conduct a basic mental state examination, in order to define straightforward abnormalities, irrespective of their diagnostic cause. Where the person's capacity is uncertain and their disabilities make the interpretation of legal tests of capacity complex, it may be appropriate to seek a specialist opinion.

15.2.1 Specialist knowledge

Hospital medicine is divided into specialities. Some patients with a possible legal incapacity require assessment by a psychiatrist, that is a medical practitioner who is trained to assess and treat disorders which may present with psychiatric or mental symptoms. Both "organically" (physically) and "functionally" (non-organically) caused illnesses can present with mental symptoms (see section 15.3.1). For example, a patient complaining of "voices" might have either schizophrenia (functional) or dementia (organic). This emphasises the importance of the primary diagnostic decision being taken by a medical practitioner (as opposed to a clinical psychologist) if there is any possibility that the condition may have an organic cause.

Once the diagnosis is clearly established as organic it may be appropriate for the patient's condition to be treated, and his or her capacity to be assessed by a non-psychiatric specialist (for example a neurologist). It is important to choose a specialist who has extensive clinical experience of the disorder and is familiar with caring for patients with that condition, rather than one having detailed research knowledge. Hence, a consultant in psychiatry of old age may be a better expert on Alzheimer's disease than a research neurologist. Since assessments of capacity have a practical purpose, they should be based on a practical knowledge of the condition and of its manifestations, treatability, and prognosis.

Many patients can be best assessed by their general practitioner. A close, long-term acquaintance between the doctor and the patient may be a major asset in creating the best environment to maximise the patient's capacity (see section 2.3). It is important, however, to emphasise that a general practitioner's close and personal knowledge of a patient, even concern and affection, must not be allowed to interfere with an objective assessment about the patient's actual mental disabilities and implied (in)capacities. Sometimes it is desirable for a general practitioner and a hospital specialist to consult together in determining their individual views of the patient's capacity. This offers the advantage of combining expertise in the management of a complicated condition with close acquaintance with the patient.

Examples of relevant specialist opinions, in relation to particular diagnoses, might be as follows:

- consultant general psychiatrist for schizophrenia, severe depressive illness, mania, paranoid psychosis
- consultant in old age psychiatry (formerly known as psychogeriatrician) for Alzheimer's disease or other dementias, or mental illness in older people
- consultant psychiatrist in learning disability for learning disability
- consultant general psychiatrist or consultant general physician with a special interest in eating disorders for anorexia nervosa and other eating disorders
- consultant neurologist or consultant neuropsychiatrist for head injury, epilepsy, multiple sclerosis
- consultant neurologist or consultant neurosurgeon for brain tumour.

15.2.2 Other disciplines

Any medical opinion should take full account of relevant information from other disciplines. An assessment by a clinical psychologist may already be available, or could be sought, and this may assist in giving a detailed, validated and systematic assessment of cognitive functioning. An occupational therapist has special skills in assessing disabilities which may interfere with activities in everyday tasks. A report from a nurse or a social worker may be helpful where information about daily activities or social functioning is of importance. What is important is not the diagnosis per se, but the specific disabilities.

15.2.3 Medicolegal expertise

In a complex medicolegal case it may be helpful for the lawyer to choose a doctor with particular experience in medicolegal work. Experience of sifting through large volumes of medical and other information and knowledge of some of the potential complexities of the interface between medicine and law can greatly assist a clear presentation of the medical issues. It is important, however, that experts are chosen primarily for their medical knowledge and not simply because they "do a lot of court work". Medical knowledge plus medicolegal experience is often a helpful combination.

15.3 Psychiatric diagnoses

15.3.1 Categories of diagnoses

Psychiatric diagnoses can be divided into those that are organic and those that are functional.

Organic conditions

Organic conditions arise from brain disorders or from some general malfunction of the body (for example, of the endocrine or hormone system). Brain disorders can be further subdivided into *acute* (for example, an acute confusional state from urinary retention or from a toxic infective cause) and *chronic* (for example, dementia). The latter is differentiated into *congenital* (for example, some forms of learning disability) or *acquired* (for example, from a head injury) types.

Functional disorders

Functional disorders are subdivided into *mental illness* (which involves a change in the person's mental state away from their usual, normal state and which can either be temporary or permanent) and *personality disorder*. Personality disorder is a general term which includes so-called "psychopathic disorders" (although there has been much debate about the useful or otherwise of that term). Psychopathy has been described as involving "deeply ingrained maladaptive patterns of behaviour, generally recognisable by the time of adolescence or earlier, and continuing throughout adult life, although becoming less obvious in middle or old age".[2] Mental illnesses can be further subdivided into those that are *psychotic* and those that are *neurotic*. Psychotic illnesses (such as schizophrenia, hypomania and psychotic depression) involve lack of insight and the experience of delusions or hallucinations (not arising from organic causes). Neurotic illnesses (including mild to moderate depression, anxiety disorders and obsessive–compulsive disorders) involve insight and often a request for treatment. A few conditions sit on the border between psychosis and neurosis. Hence, anorexia nervosa presents with a particular mix of features where there are no hallucinations and strictly no delusions, but where there is substantial distortion of body perception, and profoundly distorted forms of thinking.

In relation to mental capacity, diagnostic categories can be thought of as existing in a hierarchy. Hence:

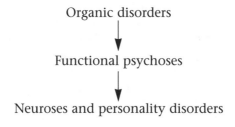

Organic disorders

Functional psychoses

Neuroses and personality disorders

It is important to note that a patient may satisfy the diagnostic criteria for more than one diagnosis. This is diagnostically acceptable but, in terms of capacity, it is likely that the disorders at the top of the hierarchy will be of greater significance.

15.3.2 Specific diagnoses

Aside from broad diagnostic categories, specific psychiatric diagnoses are made on the basis of particular clusters of symptoms and signs. Although there is a tendency for these clusters to overlap somewhat (and this can give rise to diagnostic disputes), proper concentration on specific symptoms and signs mean that this overlap is usually relatively unimportant. The broad categorical classification system given above may be of more use in suggesting capacity, or its absence, than a specific diagnosis (particularly bearing in mind the importance of attention to specific symptoms and signs in any event).

There are two accepted international systems for the classification of mental disorders, the World Health Organization's international classification of disease (WHO ICD-10) and the American Psychiatric Association's diagnostic and statistical manual (DSM-IV). It is helpful if medical reports tie the diagnosis into one of these systems to ensure diagnostic consistency between doctors.

15.4 Medical assessment of mental conditions

Although capacity may be influenced by physical conditions it is crucially important for any assessing doctor to take a full psychiatric history and to carry out a mental state examination, as well as a general medical assessment of the person. In psychiatry "symptoms" are what the patient tells you and "signs" are the doctor's objective observation of the patient. In psychiatric assessment, however, although some signs are clearly objective: a depressed patient may be dishevelled when usually well turned out. Many signs involve a medical interpretation of the patient's symptom complaints: does the patient's complaint of "voices" really amount to auditory hallucinations? Is a strange belief held with such conviction that it amounts to a delusion? Thus a degree of ambiguity can arise which is less common in other branches of medicine. It is not the case, however, that psychiatric assessments are inherently personal to the individual doctor or inherently ambiguous. High levels of diagnostic reliability should be expected.

Psychiatric assessment includes assessment for both organic and functional conditions. Hence the assessment should always include at least a brief physical assessment and, when indicated by the history or by physical observation, more detailed physical examination and investigation.

15.4.1 History

The process of psychiatric assessment involves several criteria, as described below.

History of presenting complaint

This is the description by a patient of his or her main complaints (symptoms). The doctor will pursue symptoms, by asking specific and direct questions aimed at elucidating the symptoms, specifically considering the possible differential diagnosis. Where the assessment is in relation to the patient's capacity, it may also be appropriate to pursue certain relevant symptoms in detail and to ask questions specifically relevant to the particular capacity concerned.

Background history

This includes a brief description of the patient's personal history, family history, psychosexual history (including obstetric and gynaecological history), social history, and any previous forensic history.

Pre-morbid personality

A description by the patient (or more appropriately by a relative or others) of the patient's usual personality (that is when not mentally or otherwise ill). This is important as a baseline against which the patient's current symptom complaints (and presentation at interview) can be assessed.

Previous medical history

This details all non-psychiatric conditions and treatments, including reference to any drugs that the patient is currently taking. The history may give clues as to a physical cause of apparently psychiatric symptoms.

Previous psychiatric history

This can be of relevance to current mental state assessment. A history of previous disorder may give clues about the origins of present symptoms (or signs).

Drugs and alcohol history

This may be of great relevance to the determination of the differential diagnosis of mental disorder (since drugs or chronic alcohol abuse can cause psychiatric presentations).

Information from others

This is important because patients may misrepresent symptoms (either hiding them or exaggerating them) or they may describe their usual personality in a way which is heavily influenced by their current illness (for example, depressed patients may describe themselves as being "useless" and "incapable at work" whereas the reverse may be the case). In assessing a person for some legal capacity, however, it is important to bear in mind that the person providing the information may have a vested interest (either social or financial) in the doctor's assessment of the person's capacity and care must be taken to allow for this possibility. Information from a number of people may be essential to sift out truth from bias.

15.4.2 Mental state examination

This is an objective assessment of the patient's mental functioning. The purpose of such an examination is to define specific abnormalities (and disabilities) and to establish a diagnosis. It is only through detailed assessment of specific aspects of mental functioning that capacity can properly be assessed. The following features are relevant in any assessment carried out by a doctor:

- appearance and behaviour
- speech
- mood
- thought
- perception
- cognition
- orientation
- memory
- intelligence
- insight.

An explanation of the process of the mental state examination is set out in section 14.5.

15.4.3 Physical examination

Psychiatric assessment may properly include a brief physical assessment. In some cases, where indicated by the history or by physical observation, a more detailed physical examination and investigation may be required. It is important to keep in mind that an apparent psychiatric presentation can be indicative of an organic neurological disorder and some patients can present neurologically and yet have a primary psychiatric condition (hysterical symptoms being an obvious example). The neurology of higher cortical functions and psychiatry are often intricately intertwined; conditions such as dementia are both "psychiatric" and "neurological". Many functional psychiatric conditions, such as schizophrenia, have demonstrable organic aspects and are also probably partially determined by genetic predisposition, obstetric complications, childhood infections, and perhaps other conditions affecting the brain.

15.4.4 Medical records

It is important for the assessing doctor to have access to all relevant medical and psychiatric records. These give an historical picture of a known current disorder, as well as giving diagnostic clues to a so far undiagnosed current disorder. In assessing capacity this historical view may be of particular importance, especially in relation both to the likely response to treatment and to prognosis, since these may affect future capacity. Assessment of the likely duration of disabilities may be crucially important in offering a view about capacity. These issues are especially important in cases where the legal process can be delayed. Wherever possible, priority should be given to enabling people to regain capacity and hence to retake control over their own lives.

References and notes

1 In the Estate of Park, Park v Park [1954] P 112. Masterman-Lister v Brutton & Co and Jewell & Home Counties Dairies [2003] 3 All ER 162.
2 World Health Organization. *ICD-9* (1978) cited in: Mason JK, McCall Smith RA, Laurie GT. *Law and medical ethics, 6th ed.* Edinburgh: Butterworths, 2002:652–3.

Appendices

Appendix A

Case studies

Case 1

Archie is 81 years old and was formerly a high-ranking civil servant. He now suffers from senile dementia manifested primarily by a deficit in his short-term memory. Four years ago he had two small strokes which contributed to the onset of the memory deficit. His wife, Barbara, died last year and since her death he has only been able to remain in his own home with the support of a neighbour, Connie, whom he often refers to as Barbara. His next of kin is a son who lives 200 miles away and rarely visits him. Archie has an estate worth roughly £550 000. The value of his house is about £225 000 and, although he has no mortgage, he has the usual out-goings to pay – council tax, water charges, gas, electricity, telephone and insurance – and there are his normal day-to-day living expenses. He has £75 000 in banks and building societies, and a portfolio of shares and unit trusts worth approximately £250 000. The income from his occupational pension, state pension, and investments comes to about £27 000 a year.

Archie recently wrote to his solicitor saying that he wanted help with his finances and wished to make a new will leaving a legacy of £100 000 to Connie. He also hinted that he was thinking about marrying her. With Archie's consent the solicitor contacted his GP, explained the situation, and mentioned that it would probably be necessary to carry out at least four separate assessments of capacity (spread over several visits). Archie also agreed that any confidential information about his property and affairs which might be relevant could be disclosed to his GP. The specific tests the solicitor had in mind were for:

- capacity to create an enduring power of attorney (EPA)
- capacity to manage and administer his property and affairs
- capacity to make a will
- capacity to marry.

On her first visit, the GP established that Archie was capable of creating an enduring power of attorney appointing the solicitor as attorney. Archie was capable of understanding and did understand that:

- the attorney would be able to assume complete authority over his affairs
- the attorney would in general be able to do anything with his property that he could have done personally
- the authority given under the enduring power would continue if he should be, or become, mentally incapable
- if he should be, or become, mentally incapable, he could not revoke the enduring power of attorney without confirmation by the Court of Protection.

The GP was also of the opinion that Archie was "incapable, by reason of mental disorder, of managing and administering his property and affairs". This involved establishing first that he had a "mental disorder" as defined in the Mental Health Act 1983. There was no problem here. Archie suffers from dementia, classified as a mental illness (see section 4.2.2). Secondly, the GP considered that, by reason of his mental disorder, he was or was becoming incapable of managing and administering his property and affairs.

Archie then made an EPA appointing the solicitor as his attorney. The GP witnessed Archie's execution of the power. Before executing the power the solicitor warned Archie that because the GP was of the opinion that he was incapable by reason of mental disorder of managing and administering his property and affairs, the solicitor, as attorney, would be under a duty to register the EPA with the Court of Protection straightaway. If Archie had not made, or had been incapable of making, an enduring power, someone could have applied to the Court of Protection for a person to be appointed as his receiver (see section 4.2).

Connie has been a great support to Archie during the last 12 months. Without her assistance – doing the shopping, cooking, cleaning, laundry and ironing, as well as occasional help to get washed and dressed on a bad day – it would have been impossible for him to have remained in his own home for as long as he has. His finances are potentially vulnerable, however. The phenomenon of elder abuse is not just physical, psychological, or sexual. Financial exploitation is probably the most prevalent form of elder abuse.

Archie has already bought Connie a new Ford Escort. Admittedly, he is the principal beneficiary because she spends most of her time driving him around in it. Although it cost a considerable amount, the validity of the gift is not in doubt. It was intended to be an outright gift – a token of his appreciation – and its value is insignificant in the context of his assets as a whole (see Chapter 6). He hasn't driven it yet, although, in theory, he could do so if he wanted. He still has a valid driving licence. From the age of 70 drivers have to re-apply for a licence every 3 years. When he completed the renewal application 2 years ago, he did not consider that he was suffering from any kind of mental disorder that might affect his ability to drive. The GP told the solicitor that she considers it would be unsafe for Archie to drive. Archie's solicitor informs him that he must report his illness to the Driver and Vehicle Licensing Agency who may revoke his licence. Archie agrees to do so.

Having resolved the questions of Archie's capacity to create an enduring power of attorney and manage and administer his property and affairs, the solicitor then had to deal with his ability to make a will, his "testamentary capacity". The solicitor explained to the GP that Archie should:

- understand the nature and effect of making a will
- understand the effect of the will he proposes to make
- understand the extent (rather than the actual value) of the property of which he is disposing under the will
- comprehend and appreciate the claims to which he ought to give effect.

The first three points are based on "understanding". This entails receiving, evaluating and reaching a decision on information either known to him already, or on information communicated and explained to him in broad terms and simple language by a third party, perhaps the solicitor. The final stage encompasses more than understanding – it involves Archie's judgment. He must be capable of weighing the respective merits of Connie – who he sees every day and who has been of great help to him during the last 12 months – and his son, who he rarely sees, but who is nevertheless his next of kin. This is far harder to assess because it is extremely subjective. There is also a danger that the assessor might consider Archie's decision to be foolish, but it is his capacity – rather than his wisdom – that is being assessed. Furthermore, being able to comprehend and appreciate the claims to which he ought to give effect is something that Archie must be capable of doing without help from anyone else.

The GP had to admit that she found it impossible to decide whether Archie has testamentary capacity. The solicitor therefore contacted a clinical psychologist who had assessed Archie's memory problems a couple of years ago. The clinical psychologist spent an hour and a half assessing his testamentary capacity, and was able to re-administer a couple of the tests from the earlier assessment (see section 14.5.1). He concluded that on the balance of probabilities Archie had testamentary capacity, despite his short-term memory deficit. Therefore, a will was prepared in accordance with the instructions originally contained in the letter to the solicitor, which Archie had subsequently confirmed in his conversations with those assessing his testamentary capacity. The GP and the clinical psychologist were asked to act as witnesses when Archie signed the will because of the so-called "golden – if tactless – rule" that "when a solicitor is drawing up a will for an aged testator or one who has been seriously ill, it should be witnessed or approved by a medical practitioner, who ought to record his examination of the testator and his findings" (see sections 3.5 and 5.4).

If it had been decided that on the balance of probabilities Archie lacked testamentary capacity, the solicitor would have considered applying to the Court of Protection for an order under the Mental Health Act 1983 authorising the execution of a statutory will on his behalf (see section 5.7). Because such an application would have been made on behalf of the donor of a registered enduring power of attorney, the court would have required medical evidence of both (a) his testamentary capacity, and (b) his capacity to manage and administer his property and affairs. If it had been necessary to apply for a statutory will, Archie's son would have been given notice of the application by the court. But because Archie was capable of making a valid will for himself, the solicitor had no obligation to inform the son about the changes his father proposed to make to his will. Indeed, to have told the son would have constituted a breach of the solicitor's duty to keep a client's affairs confidential until the client permits disclosure or waives confidentiality (see section 2.2.1).

The final type of capacity to be assessed is whether Archie is capable of entering into a valid marriage (see section 10.4). There is an additional complication here. A will is automatically revoked when the person who made it gets married, unless the will was specifically expressed to be made in expectation of that marriage. Archie and Connie are not engaged and at the moment have no definite plans to marry. The will was not, therefore, expressed to be made in expectation of their forthcoming marriage. If Archie does eventually marry Connie, a further assessment of testamentary capacity will be necessary. If it is concluded that he lacks testamentary capacity at that time, an application could be made to the Court of Protection for the execution of a statutory will. If he still has testamentary capacity he could, of course, make a valid will for himself.

It has been suggested that the capacity required to enter into a valid marriage is relatively low. If Archie and Connie decide to get married, it will be necessary to establish at the time the decision is made whether he is capable of giving valid consent (and that, for instance, she is not pressurising him into marrying her against his will), and that he understands the nature of marriage and respective rights and responsibilities of husband and wife. Their friendship has allegedly assumed a sexual dimension, but his capacity to consent to sexual relations is not an issue (see section 10.3).

Case 2

John is in his late 60s and has been diagnosed as suffering from chronic schizophrenia. He has delusions that people are interfering with his thoughts and that they are also trying to harm him. John has developed an acute infection in his leg which is life-threatening. It is explained to him that if he does not have the leg removed there is a high probability that he will die. John refuses consent to the surgery but says he will accept the alternative of antibiotics, even intravenously. It is unlikely that this action will substantially reduce the risk of death, certainly in the medium term and perhaps even immediately. What are the possible medicolegal implications of this clinical situation?

Nothing would be gained by detaining John under mental health legislation. The law allows compulsory treatment in certain circumstances, but only for mental disorders, or their consequences. John suffers from a physical condition which is unrelated to his mental state and psychiatric diagnosis. Hence, only common law provisions are relevant.

A diagnosis of schizophrenia does not automatically imply a lack of capacity to consent to or refuse consent to treatment at common law. What matters is the nature of a person's mental state abnormalities and how they relate to the definition in law of capacity, that is, the ability to comprehend and retain the information material to the decision, especially with respect to the consequences of having or not having the treatment in question, and to use the information and weigh it in the balance as part of the process of arriving at a decision (see section 12.3). Only if a patient lacks capacity according to this definition can the common law be invoked so as to treat the patient without consent.

Much more needs to be known about John's psychiatric symptoms than has been described so far before a conclusion about his capacity can be reached. If, for example, he had incorporated the treatment information and/or the healthcare personnel into his paranoid delusions then – although this may not interfere with his capacity to receive and retain the treatment information (and information about the consequences of non-treatment) – it may well inhibit or impair his capacity to "weigh" up that information to come to a decision. If, on the other hand, the delusions were unconnected with the treatment information and the medical personnel, and therefore not connected to his decision about surgical treatment, John would have capacity to refuse consent.

If, however, John later became septicemic (from the local infection) then, at that point, any cognitive abnormality arising from an acute state of confusion might well result in a lack of capacity. He could then be treated under the doctrine of necessity in his best interests (see section 12.4). However, if John had either (a) previously obtained a court declaration that he then had capacity to refuse the treatment and that the procedure should not be carried out without his consent, or (b) made an "advance directive" (see section 12.5.2) that he could not be treated without his consent in the future, then even the supervening acute confusional state (and lack of capacity) would fail to render lawful the surgical intervention – so long as it was for the same physical condition and in circumstances John had foreseen. John could, of course, revoke the effect of the advance directive in the future so long as he had the capacity to do so.

If John subsequently had a stroke, having thus far survived the local infection, then specific cognitive abnormalities might interfere with his capacity to receive and/or retain treatment information, and depending on the area of the brain affected by the stroke, this might affect his capacity to weigh that information. Alternatively, it might give rise to a disability whereby John became limited in verbal expression (for example, nominal aphasia). If so, every effort should be made to limit the impact of such communication difficulties, rather than to equate them with incapacity. In the event that capacity was significantly impaired and John had already made an advance directive whilst competent, the directive would be effective notwithstanding the supervening incapacity. John's earlier refusal could not be overridden and he would have lost the capacity to revoke the original advance directive. If, however, a different physical condition arose which was not covered by the advance directive, then the doctrine of necessity could justify treatment for that condition without consent (if John now lacked capacity). Indeed any treatment of the stroke itself could be carried out under the same principle.

Case 3

Jane is 19 years old and has Down syndrome. When she was 11 years old her mother died and Jane was placed by her father into the care of the local social services authority. She lived with several foster families for short periods but was finally permanently placed with a family at the age of 13. Until she was 18 Jane lived with this family under the provisions of a Residence Order obtained as a result of proceedings brought under the Children Act 1989. During this period Jane continued to see her father during occasional weekends and had contact with him through letters and telephone calls.

When Jane became 18 she was entitled as an adult to decide where she wished to live. She was very clear that she wished to continue to live with her present family, which is a large extended family caring for other children and young adults with learning disabilities. Shortly after her 18th birthday Jane became engaged to marry a man she met on her college course. This man also had Down syndrome and her father disapproved of the relationship. He asked Jane to return to live with him and his second wife, which would take her away from her fiancé. Jane was adamant that she wanted to stay put and her refusal caused conflict between her father and her current carers and family. Jane became very upset and distressed by this and by her father's continued contact, which she said had become unpleasant. She stated that she no longer wished to see her father at all or have any phone calls or letters from him. Jane has the right to decide about her own family relationships and no-one can force her to continue contact with her father (see section 10.2). Subsequent to this Jane married her husband (her capacity to consent to marriage was not questioned – see section 10.4) and they both remain living in independent accommodation within the extended family home. They have no contact with Jane's father but have regular contact with her husband's family, which is positive and supportive.

Jane's father then started proceedings in the Family Division of the High Court to ask the court to make a declaration as to where Jane should live, and that it would be in her best interests to have contact with him. Jane continued to say that she does not wish to have contact with her father or his family and that she wished to continue to live where she was.

Jane subsequently instructed her own solicitor. The solicitor met with Jane on a number of occasions both in her own home and in the solicitor's office and came to the conclusion that Jane had capacity to make the decision to continue to live in her present home. The solicitor also felt that Jane understood the solicitor's role, and was able to give instructions about the line to take when writing to her father's solicitors or speaking on her behalf (see section 2.1). Jane also has an advocate who meets with Jane and her solicitor to assist Jane in representing her views to the solicitor.

Despite attempts at negotiation through the solicitors, the court proceedings are to continue. The first stage of the proceedings involves consideration by the court as to whether Jane does in fact have capacity to instruct her solicitor and to participate in the legal proceedings (see Chapter 7). If the court decides on the basis of expert reports that Jane does not have capacity to manage and administer her property and affairs (in this case, the legal proceedings) and therefore instruct her solicitor, then the court would appoint a litigation friend to instruct the solicitor acting on Jane's behalf (see section 7.4). Given that Jane's husband also has learning disabilities and other people who have a close relationship with her are involved in the case, they may not be suitable to act as litigation friend, so it may be advisable to ask the Official Solicitor to take on this role (see Appendix B). After hearing all the evidence, the court will then make a declaration about where Jane should live and who she should have contact with, basing the decision on what it considers to be in her best interests. If it is found that Jane does have capacity to make these decisions for herself, the court has no jurisdiction to intervene.

There are other issues in Jane's life in which her capacity is also being questioned. Her father is considering challenging her marriage on the grounds that she had no capacity to consent to the marriage (see section 10.4). He has also raised concerns about Jane's ability to manage her money and affairs and whether someone should be appointed to do this for her (see Chapter 4).

Jane's ability to make decisions on each of these issues must be decided using a different test of capacity. Medical evidence is conflicting and it may be necessary to present more detailed evidence about Jane's day-to-day understanding of her world, in particular her ability to function on a range of tasks and skills. Jane is a vulnerable person and is susceptible to influence by others. It is very important to make sure that her decisions are, as far as possible, made voluntarily by her, with the benefit of advice and support from others as appropriate. It is, of course, very difficult for any person to make a decision that is independent of the views of others with whom the person lives or has relationships. This case presents a dilemma: to ensure high quality of care and protection for an individual who is vulnerable and who has impaired capacity in certain tasks, but who wishes to maintain her independence and decision making capacity to the maximum extent possible.

Case 4

Michael is 29 years old and suffers from severe brain damage sustained in a road accident when he was 18 years old. Until the accident he lived with his mother, step-father, brother and step-sister. He left school at 16 and became a trainee chef and was successful in his career. Immediately after the accident Michael was cared for in an acute neurological ward where he was severely ill and spent much of the time in a coma. He gradually recovered consciousness and was transferred to a rehabilitation hospital where planning for his future care began.

Michael's parents had divorced when Michael was 10 and his mother had obtained custody of Michael and his brother. The divorce had been acrimonious. Between the ages of 11 and 19, Michael had seen his father very rarely. His father had moved away and maintained only occasional contact with his two sons.

When Michael was receiving treatment at the rehabilitation hospital all his family, including his father and step-mother, visited regularly. There were clinical meetings to discuss Michael's discharge and it was always planned that he would return home to live with his mother and step-father. That way he could continue to have contact with old friends. While Michael was in hospital there was conflict between his mother and father. Subsequently Michael's father came to the hospital and removed him, taking him to live at home with him and his second wife.

Michael's mother consulted a solicitor and was informed that there was nothing she could do and that she should try to sort this out with Michael's father. The father refused to talk about Michael's future and certainly did not wish Michael to return home to live with his mother. His father maintained that this was what Michael would have wanted. Michael continued to live with his father and step-mother and to attend a day centre for head-injured patients near their home.

Eventually, on the advice of another solicitor, Michael's mother commenced proceedings in the High Court to ask the court to make a declaration as to Michael's best interests with regard to increasing contact with her and the rest of his family and as to where he should live in the future.

At present the daily care of Michael currently rests with his father and step-mother and they make most of his day-to-day decisions. Michael is unable to initiate contact with his mother by telephone, by letter, or by actively going to see her. The current issue is whether Michael is able to make the decision about whether he wishes to see his mother. His father maintains that Michael does not wish to have contact with his family and that Michael is able to make this decision.

After Michael's accident, solicitors acting on his behalf instituted a damages claim and a large award of damages was subsequently made. His affairs are managed by the Court of Protection and a solicitor was appointed as his receiver (see section 4.2). Despite this, Michael may be able to make his own decisions about other matters, including whether to see his mother, and whether he wishes to live with his mother or his father. Medical opinions are being sought to assess the degree of Michael's brain damage and psychological evidence is being sought to assess his understanding of his world and where he lives. Any decision about Michael's capacity will be based on specific situations about which he is asked to make decisions. There is a legal structure to enable others to make financial decisions on his behalf, but no legal structure to enable others to make personal decisions on his behalf. Michael's life is currently affected by those around him, in particular by his father and step-mother who live with him on a daily basis and who, at the moment, control much of his personal life.

Appendix B

The Official Solicitor

The Official Solicitor performs a wide range of duties including the representation of persons under a legal disability due to minority or mental disorder where there is no other suitable person willing and able to act. The bulk of this workload consists of representing adults who lack capacity in a wide range of litigation. This includes divorce, Family Law Act injunctions and every type of civil litigation (see Chapters 7 and 10), representing patients in the Court of Protection upon the consideration of applications for a statutory will to be made on their behalf under the Mental Health Act 1983 (see section 5.7) or for other financial transactions to be entered into on their behalf (see Chapter 4). The Official Solicitor may also act on behalf of children and young people in certain circumstances although, in general, proceedings involving children and young people under 18 years are dealt with by the Children and Family Court Advisory and Support Service (CAFCASS). The role of CAFCASS is outside the scope of this book.

Perhaps the Official Solicitor's best known role is that of guardian ad litem in proceedings where a declaration is sought as to whether proposed medical treatment or other arrangements are in the best interests of a patient.[1] The Official Solicitor is usually involved in all cases in which the giving or withholding of consent to medical treatment on behalf of an incapacitated adult patient is an issue (see section 12.4).

Whatever the type of proceedings, in order for the Official Solicitor to become involved the person who is the subject of the proceedings must be shown to be a "patient" within the meaning of Part VII of the Mental Health Act 1983, that is an adult who is incapable, by reason of mental disorder, of managing and administering his or her property and affairs (see section 7.2). Medical evidence (from a medical practitioner or psychologist) is usually required before the Official Solicitor can consent to act. The standard form of medical certificate is set out at Appendix E.

There are therefore a number of potential roles for the Official Solicitor according to the type of proceedings and the circumstances of the particular case. This may be to be the litigation friend or guardian ad litem of the person who is the subject of the proceedings (see Chapter 7). Alternatively, the role may be to obtain evidence, usually medical evidence, and instruct counsel to assist the court in the role of advocate to the court (formerly known as "amicus"). In addition the Official Solicitor may be a defendant in his or her own right, for example where otherwise the proceedings would be without a defendant. The Official Solicitor always carries out impartial and independent enquiries to ensure that all relevant information is before the court and all views are aired and expressed. When acting as litigation friend, next friend or guardian ad litem for a person under incapacity, the role of the Official Solicitor is to select and instruct solicitors as necessary, and make all the decisions required in the course of the litigation, including whether to pursue, withdraw, or settle the proceedings. While the Official Solicitor will, where possible, ascertain the views of the patient or child, and relay them to the court, he or she is not bound to follow those views but must act in the client's best interests. Independent psychiatric and other medical evidence is frequently commissioned.

The Official Solicitor's functions and duties are more fully described in Practice Notes covering declaratory proceedings relating to medical and welfare decisions[2] and family proceedings[3] which are set out in Appendix C and Appendix D. Note also the Direction issued by the President of the Family Division[4] confirming that declaratory proceedings concerning the best interests of incapacitated adults are civil proceedings and are more suitable for hearing in the Family Division than any other division of the High Court. Cases which also require the review of a decision by a public authority through judicial review proceedings in the Administrative Court, however, should preferably be heard before a nominated judge of the Administrative Court who is also a judge of the Family Division.[5]

Early contact with lawyers in the Office of the Official Solicitor is advisable in those cases in which they are to be involved. Members of staff are always prepared to discuss cases over the telephone and give general advice. The address and telephone number are listed on page 221.

Out of hours applications to court

All cases in which the giving or withholding of consent to medical treatment is an issue are heard by judges in the Family Division of the High Court. Outside normal office hours contact should be made, normally by counsel (or solicitor with higher advocacy rights), with the security officer at the Royal Courts of Justice in London. He or she contacts the designated urgent business officer by telephone, whose responsibility it is to assess the urgency of the application and, if appropriate, to contact the Duty Judge. The judge would, if necessary, contact the Official Solicitor. The judge may grant the order sought over the telephone or may direct attendance at his or her lodgings. In the event of a medicolegal emergency, it is therefore prudent to have available to speak to the judge both counsel and a relevant medical expert. A contact telephone number for the Royal Courts of Justice is given on page 222.

References and notes

1   For a more detailed description of the court's role and the involvement of the Official Solicitor in medical treatment decisions, see: Oates L. The court's role in decisions about medical treatment. *BMJ* 2000;**321**:1282–4. Further information is available at http://www.offsol.demon.co.uk.
2   Practice Note (Official Solicitor: Declaratory Proceedings: Medical and Welfare Decisions for Adults who Lack Capacity) [2001] 2 FLR 158.
3   Practice Note (Official Solicitor: Appointment in Family Proceedings) [2001] 2 FLR 155.
4   Practice Direction (Declaratory Proceedings: Incapacitated Adults) [2002] 1 All ER 794.
5   A v A Health Authority and another; In re J (A Child) [2002] Fam 213.

Appendix C

Practice Note

Official Solicitor: Declaratory Proceedings: Medical And Welfare Decisions For Adults Who Lack Capacity

1 This practice note supersedes practice notes dated June 1996 (Official Solicitor: Sterilisation [1996] 2 FLR 111) and July 1996 (Official Solicitor: Vegetative state [1996] 2 FLR 375). It combines the guidance given in those earlier practice notes, and extends it to a wider range of medical and welfare disputes leading to litigation. This practice note deals only with adults who lack capacity. Medical treatment or welfare disputes about children will be dealt with under the Children Act 1989 or the inherent jurisdiction in relation to children (see practice notes: Official Solicitor: Appointment in Family Proceedings [2001] Fam Law 307; and Officers of CAFCASS Legal Services and Special Casework: Appointment in Family Proceedings [2001] Fam Law 249).

Jurisdiction

2 The High Court has jurisdiction to make declarations as to the best interests of an adult who lacks decision-making capacity. The jurisdiction will be exercised when there is a serious justiciable issue requiring a decision by the court. It has been exercised in relation to a range of medical treatment issues, in particular sterilisation operations and the continuance of artificial nutrition and hydration. It has also been exercised in relation to residence and contact issues. The jurisdiction is comprehensively reviewed and analysed in *Re F (Adult: Court's Jurisdiction)* [2000] 2 FLR 512.

The need for court involvement

3 Case law has established two categories of case that will in virtually all cases require the prior sanction of a High Court

judge. The first is sterilisation of a person (whether a child or an adult) who cannot consent to the operation: *Re B (A Minor) (Wardship: Sterilisation)* [1988] AC 199 and *Re F (Mental Patient: Sterilisation)* [1990] 2 AC 1. The second is the discontinuance of artificial nutrition and hydration for a patient in a vegetative state: *Airedale NHS Trust v Bland* [1993] AC 789, 805. Further guidance about sterilisation and vegetative state cases is given below. In all other cases, doctors and carers should seek advice from their own lawyers about the need to apply to the court. In the Official Solicitor's view, applications should be made where there are disputes or difficulties as to either the patient's capacity or the patient's best interests. Guidelines were handed down by the Court of Appeal in *St George's Healthcare NHS Trust v S; R v Collins and Others ex parte S* [1998] 2 FLR 728, 758–760. It was stressed in that case that a declaration made without notice would be ineffective and ought not to be made.

The application

4   Applications should be made to the Family Division of the High Court (principal or district registry). The proceedings are not, however, "family proceedings" for the purposes of Civil Procedure Rules 1998, r2.1(2). The Civil Procedure Rules will therefore apply.

The claim

5   In the Official Solicitor's view, the Part 8 alternative procedure is the more appropriate and a Part 8 claim form should be used. The claimant should file all evidence with the claim form. The Official Solicitor is unlikely to be in a position to file all his evidence with his acknowledgment of service. A directions hearing should therefore be fixed when the claim form is issued.

6   The relief sought should be declarations that (see appendices below for suggested wording in sterilisation and PVS cases):

1. [The patient] lacks capacity to make a decision about ... [specify treatment or welfare decision at issue, for example, "having a kidney transplant" or "where to live"].

2. It is [or is not] in the existing circumstances in the best interests of [the patient] for ... [specify treatment or other issue, for example, "him to undergo below-knee amputation of his left leg" or "her to have contact with the claimant for at least 2 hours each week"].

The evidence

7 The claimant must adduce evidence going to both capacity and best interests.

1. *Capacity* The court has no jurisdiction unless it is established that the patient is incapable of making a decision about the matter in issue. The test of capacity to consent to or refuse treatment is set out in *Re MB (Medical Treatment)* [1997] 2 FLR 426, 437. In the Official Solicitor's view, this test can be used for a wide range of decisions. Evidence from a psychiatrist or psychologist who has assessed the patient applying the *Re MB* test to the particular decision in question is generally required. It follows from the terms of the *Re MB* test that global psychometric test results are unlikely to be relevant. The Official Solicitor's experience is that references to the outdated and discredited concept of "mental age" are of no assistance at all. It is important for the expert assessing capacity to advise whether the patient is likely to develop capacity to make personal decisions about the matter in issue in the future.

2. *Best interests* In any medical case, the claimant must adduce evidence from a responsible medical practitioner not only (1) that performing the particular operation would not be negligent but also (2) that it is necessary in the best interests of the patient: *Re A (Male Sterilisation)* [2000] 1 FLR 549, 555. The court's jurisdiction is to declare the best interests of the patient on the application of a welfare test analogous to that applied in wardship: *Re S (Sterilisation: Patient's Best Interests)* [2000] 2 FLR 389, 403. The judicial decision will incorporate broader ethical, social, moral and welfare considerations (ibid, 401). Emotional, psychological and social benefit to the patient will be

considered: *Re Y (Mental Patient: Bone Marrow Transplant)* [1997] Fam 110. The court will wish to prepare a balance sheet listing the advantages and disadvantages of the procedure for the patient. If potential advantages and disadvantages are to be relied on then the court will wish to assess in percentage terms the likelihood of them in fact occurring: *Re A (Male Sterilisation)* [2000] 1 FLR 549, 560.

The parties

8 The claimant should be the NHS Trust or other body responsible for the patient's care, although a claim may also be brought by a family member or other individual closely connected with the patient. The body with clinical or caring responsibility should in any event be made a party: *Re S (Hospital Patient: Court's Jurisdiction)* [1996] Fam 1.

9 The person concerned must always be a party and should normally be a defendant, with the Official Solicitor acting as litigation friend. The Official Solicitor has a standard form of medical certificate if there is any question about whether the person concerned is a "patient" within the meaning of Civil Procedure Rules 1998, r21. If the Official Solicitor does not act as litigation friend, the court will wish to consider whether he should be joined as an ex officio defendant or invited to act as a friend of the court. The Official Solicitor is invariably asked to be involved in sterilisation and vegetative state cases.

The directions hearing

10 Unless the matter is urgent, the claimant should fix a directions hearing for no less than 8 weeks after the date of issue, to allow the Official Solicitor to make initial enquiries. The court should, if appropriate, be asked to hold the directions hearing in private to protect the interests of the patient: Civil Procedure Rules 1998, r39.2(3)(d). The court will use the directions hearing to:

1. make orders where necessary to preserve the anonymity of the patient, family and other parties;

2. set a timetable for the Official Solicitor to conduct enquiries, obtain expert evidence and file his statement or report;

3. fix a further hearing, to serve either as a final hearing if the matter is unopposed or as a final directions hearing to fix a contested hearing.

The Official Solicitor's enquiries

11 The Official Solicitor's representative will always see the patient, review relevant medical/social work records and interview carers, family members and others close to the patient as appropriate.

12 The Official Solicitor will consider the patient's wishes and feelings, and will enquire as to any earlier views the patient may have expressed, either in writing or otherwise. The High Court may determine the effect of a purported advance statement as to future medical treatment: *Re T (Adult: Refusal of Medical Treatment)* [1993] Fam 95, *Re C (Adult: Refusal of Medical Treatment)* [1994] 1 WLR 290. A valid and applicable advance refusal of treatment may be determinative. Previously expressed wishes and feelings which do not amount to an effective advance decision will still be an important component in the best interests decision.

The final hearing

13 Any substantive hearing should be before a High Court judge of the Family Division. Cases proceeding unopposed may be disposed of without oral evidence. The final hearing may be in private if necessary to protect the interests of the patient: Civil Procedure Rules 1998, r39.2(3)(d). If the hearing is in public, there may be orders that the identities of parties and witnesses (other than expert witnesses) should not be disclosed: Civil Procedure Rules 1998, r39.2(4). An order restricting publicity will continue to have effect notwithstanding the death of the patient, unless and until an application is made to discharge it: *Re C (Adult Patient: Publicity)* [1996] 2 FLR 251. The Official Solicitor will invite the court to make an appropriate order in relation to his costs.

Consultation with the Official Solicitor

14 Members of the Official Solicitor's legal staff are prepared to discuss adult medical and welfare cases before proceedings are issued. Enquiries should be addressed to a family litigation lawyer at:

The Official Solicitor
81 Chancery Lane
London WC2A 1DD
Telephone: 020 7911 7127
Fax: 020 7911 7105
email: enquiries@offsol.gsi.gov.uk

Enquiries about **children** medical and welfare cases should be directed to:

CAFCASS Legal Services and Special Casework
Newspaper House
8–16 Great New Street
London EC4A 3BN
Telephone: 020 7904 0867
Fax: 020 7904 0868/9
email: legal@cafcass.gsi.gov.uk

Staff of CAFCASS Legal will liaise with the Official Solicitor where it is unclear which office can best represent a child.

Laurence Oates,Official Solicitor
1 May 2001

Appendix 1: Sterilisation cases

1 If a sterilisation procedure is necessary for therapeutic as opposed to contraceptive purposes then there may be no need for an application to court: *Re GF (Medical Treatment)* [1992] 1 FLR 293. If, however, any case lies anywhere near the boundary line it should be referred to the court: *Re S (Sterilisation)* [2000] 2 FLR 389, 405.

The claim

2 The relief sought in relation to an adult should be declarations that:

1. [The patient] lacks capacity to consent to an operation of … [specify procedure proposed, for example, "tubal occlusion by Filshie clips", or "laparoscopic sub-total hysterectomy", or "vasectomy"].
2. It is in the existing circumstances in the best interests of [the patient] for her/him to undergo an operation of … [specify procedure as above].

The evidence

3 The court must be satisfied that the patient lacks capacity and that the operation will promote the best interests of the patient, rather than the interests or convenience of the claimant, carers or public. In sterilisation cases, the best interests tests has at least three particular components:

1. *Likelihood of pregnancy*: An operation must address a current real need. It must be shown that the patient is capable of conception and is having or is likely to have full sexual intercourse. In relation to a young woman who has no interest in human relationships with any sexual ingredient a high level of supervision is an appropriate protection: *Re LC (Medical Treatment) (Sterilisation)* [1997] *2 FLR 258*. Any risk of pregnancy should be identifiable rather than speculative: *Re S (Medical Treatment: Adult Sterilisation)* [1998] *1 FLR 944*.
2. *Damage deriving from conception and/or menstruation*: The physical and psychological consequences of pregnancy and childbirth for the patient should be analysed by obstetric and psychiatric experts. In the case of a male, these considerations will be different: *Re A (Male Sterilisation)* [2000] *1 FLR 549, 557*. Psychiatric evidence as to the patient's likely ability to care for and/or have a fulfilling relationship with a child should be adduced. Evidence as to any child having a disability is likely to be irrelevant: *Re X (Adult Sterilisation)* [1998] *2 FLR 1124, 1129*. If the proposed procedure is intended to affect the patient's menstruation, then evidence about any detriment caused by her current menstrual cycle must also be adduced.
3. *Medical and surgical techniques*: The court will require a detailed analysis of all available and relevant methods of addressing any problems found to be substantiated

under (1) and (2) above. This analysis should be performed by a doctor or doctors with expertise in the full range of available methods. The expert should explain the nature of each relevant method and then list its advantages and disadvantages (in particular, morbidity rates, mortality rates and failure rates) for the individual patient, taking into account any relevant aspects of her physical and psychological health. The Royal College of Obstetrics and Gynaecology has published relevant evidence-based clinical guidelines (No 4: *Male and Female Sterilisation*, April 1999 and No 5: *The Management of Menorrhagia in Secondary Care*, July 1999).

Appendix 2: Permanent vegetative state cases

1   It is futile to provide medical treatment, including artificial nutrition and hydration, to a patient with no awareness of self or environment and no prospect of recovery: *Airedale NHS Trust v Bland* [1993] AC 789, 869. The purpose of the proceedings is to establish whether the patient is in this condition. It is not appropriate to apply to court to discontinue artificial feeding and hydration until the condition is judged to be permanent. Diagnostic guidelines are not statutory provisions and a precise label may not be of importance. The court's concern is whether there is any awareness whatsoever or any possibility of change: *Re D (Medical Treatment)* [1998] 1 FLR 411, 420 and *Re H (A Patient)* [1998] 2 FLR 36. The approach of the court has been reviewed in the light of the Human Rights Act 1998 and held to be compatible with Convention rights: *NHS Trust A v M: NHS Trust B v H* [2001] 1 FCR 406. There has as yet been no decided case dealing with the discontinuance of artificial feeding and hydration for an adult patient with any (however minimal) awareness of self or environment.

The claim

2   All claims in these cases should be issued in the Principal Registry and will normally be heard by the President of the Family Division unless she releases the case to another Family Division judge. The relief sought should be declarations that:

1. [The patient] lacks capacity to consent to continued life-sustaining treatment measures and is in the permanent vegetative state.
2. It is not in the existing circumstances in the best interests of [the patient] to be given life-sustaining medical treatment measures (including ventilation, nutrition and hydration by artificial means) and such measures may lawfully be discontinued.
3. It is in [the patient's] best interests to be given such treatment and nursing care whether at hospital or elsewhere under medical supervision as may be appropriate to ensure he/she retains the greatest dignity until such time as his/her life comes to an end.

The medical evidence

3   The diagnosis should be made in accordance with the most up-to-date generally accepted guidelines for the medical profession. A review by a working group of the Royal College of Physicians has been endorsed by the Conference of Medical Royal Colleges (*The Permanent Vegetative State*, Royal College of Physicians Publication Unit, 1996; with addendum published in *J R Coll Physicians* (1997) 31, 260). The review concludes that the diagnosis of permanent vegetative state should not be made until the patient has been in a continuing vegetative state following head injury for 12 months or following other causes of brain damage for 6 months. The addendum to the review emphasises that there is no urgency in making the diagnosis and the assessors should take into account descriptions given by relatives, carers and nursing staff who spend most time with the patient. The *International Working Party Report on the Vegetative State* (1996), produced by the Royal Hospital for Neuro-disability, sets out in an appendix a range of vegetative presentations.

4   The claimant should, as a minimum, adduce evidence from (1) the treating physician and (2) a neurologist or other expert experienced in assessing disturbances of consciousness. Both should deal with the diagnosis and their professional judgment of whether continued treatment would be in the patient's best interests. The duties of doctors making the diagnosis are described in the Royal College of Physicians review.

5   The court will generally wish to see at least two reports from experts, one of whom must be independent of the treating clinical team and claimant. The Official Solicitor will usually commission the second expert report.

Other evidence

6   The claimant should also adduce evidence about the views of family members. The views of family members or others close to the patient cannot act as a veto to an application but they must be taken fully into account by the court: *Re G (Persistent Vegetative State)* [1995] 2 FCR 46, 51.

The final hearing

7   It is usual for the final hearing to be in public, with protection for the identities of parties and witnesses. Even if the matter is unopposed, it may be appropriate for at least one expert to attend to give oral evidence. Family members need not attend if this would cause distress.

Appendix D

Practice Note

Official Solicitor: Appointment in Family Proceedings

1 This Practice Note supersedes the Practice Note dated 4 December 1998 (Official Solicitor: Appointment in Family Proceedings [1999] 1 FLR 310) issued by the Official Solicitor in relation to his appointment in family proceedings. It is issued in conjunction with a Practice Note dealing with the appointment of Officers of CAFCASS Legal Services and Special Casework in family proceedings. This Practice Note is intended to be helpful guidance, but always subject to Practice Directions, decisions of the court and other legal guidance.

2 The Children and Family Court Advisory and Support Service (CAFCASS) has responsibilities in relation to children in family proceedings in which their welfare is or may be in question (Criminal Justice and Court Services Act 2000, section 12). From 1 April 2001 the Official Solicitor will no longer represent children who are the subject of family proceedings (other than in very exceptional circumstances and after liaison with CAFCASS).

3 This Practice Note summarises the continuing role of the Official Solicitor in family proceedings. Since there are no provisions for parties under disability in the Family Proceedings Courts (Children Act 1989) Rules 1991, the Official Solicitor can only act in the High Court or in a county court, pursuant to Part IX of Family Proceedings Rules 1991. The Official Solicitor will shortly issue an updated Practice Note about his role for adults under disability who are the subject of declaratory proceedings in relation to their medical treatment or welfare.

Adults under disability

4 The Official Solicitor will, in the absence of any other willing and suitable person, act as next friend or guardian

ad litem of an adult party under disability, a "patient". "Patient" means someone who is incapable by reason of mental disorder of managing and administering his property and affairs (Family Proceedings Rules 1991, rule 9.1). Medical evidence will usually be required before the Official Solicitor can consent to act and his staff can provide a standard form of medical certificate. Where there are practical difficulties in obtaining such medical evidence, the Official Solicitor should be consulted.

Non-subject children

5 Again in the absence of any other willing and suitable person, the Official Solicitor will act as next friend or guardian ad litem of a child party whose own welfare is not the subject of family proceedings (Family Proceedings Rules 1991, r2.57, r9.2 and r9.5). The most common examples will be:

(a) a child who is also the parent of a child, and who is a respondent to a Children Act or Adoption Act application. If a child respondent is already represented by a CAFCASS officer in pending proceedings of which he or she is the subject, then the Official Solicitor will liaise with CAFCASS to agree the most appropriate arrangements;

(b) a child who wishes to make an application for a Children Act order naming another child (typically a contact order naming a sibling). The Official Solicitor will need to satisfy himself that the proposed proceedings would benefit the child applicant before proceeding;

(c) a child witness to some disputed factual issue in a children case and who may require intervener status. In such circumstances the need for party status and legal representation should be weighed in the light of *Re H (Care Proceedings: Intervener)* [2000] 1 FLR 775;

(d) a child party to a petition for a declaration of status under Part III of the Family Law Act 1986;

(e) a child intervener in divorce or ancillary relief proceedings (r2.57 or r9.5);

(f) a child applicant for, or respondent to, an application for an order under Part IV of the Family Law Act 1996.

In the case of a child applicant, the Official Solicitor will need to satisfy himself that the proposed proceedings would benefit the child before pursuing them, with leave under Family Law Act 1996, section 43 if required.

6   Any children who are parties to Children Act or inherent jurisdiction proceedings may rely on the provisions of Family Proceedings Rules 1991 rule 9.2A if they wish to instruct a solicitor without the intervention of a next friend or guardian ad litem. Rule 9.2A does not apply to Adoption Act 1976, Family Law Act 1996 or Matrimonial Causes Act 1973 proceedings.

Older children who are also patients

7   Officers of CAFCASS will not be able to represent anyone who is over the age of 18. The Official Solicitor may therefore be the more appropriate next friend or guardian ad litem of a child who is also a patient and whose disability will persist beyond his or her 18th birthday, especially in non-emergency cases where the substantive hearing is unlikely to take place before the child's 18th birthday. The Official Solicitor may also be the more appropriate next friend or guardian ad litem in medical treatment cases such as sterilisation or vegetative state cases, in which his staff have particular expertise deriving from their continuing role for adult patients.

Advising the court

8   The Official Solicitor may be invited to act or instruct counsel as a friend of the court (amicus) if it appears to the court that such an invitation is more appropriately addressed to him rather than (or in addition to) CAFCASS Legal Services and Special Casework.

Liaison with CAFCASS

9   In cases of doubt or difficulty, staff of the Official Solicitor's office will liaise with staff of CAFCASS Legal Services and Special Casework to avoid duplication and ensure the most suitable arrangements are made.

Invitations to act in new cases

10 Solicitors who have been consulted by a child or an adult under disability (or by someone acting on their behalf, or concerned about their interests) should write to the Official Solicitor setting out the background to the proposed case and explaining why there is no other willing and suitable person to act as next friend or guardian ad litem. Where the person concerned is an adult, medical evidence in the standard form of the Official Solicitor's medical certificate should be provided.

Invitations to act in pending proceedings

11 Where a case is already before the court, an order appointing the Official Solicitor should be expressed as being made subject to his consent. The Official Solicitor aims to provide a response to any invitation within 10 working days. He will be unable to consent to act for an adult until satisfied that the party is a "patient". A further directions appointment after 28 days may therefore be helpful. If he accepts appointment the Official Solicitor will need time to prepare the case on behalf of the child or patient and may wish to make submissions about any substantive hearing date. The following documents should be forwarded to the Official Solicitor without delay:

(a) a copy of the order inviting him to act (with a note of the reasons approved by the judge if appropriate);
(b) the court file;
(c) if available, a bundle with summary, statement of issues and chronology (as required by President's Direction of 10 March 2000).

Contacting the Official Solicitor

12 It is often helpful to discuss the question of appointment with the Official Solicitor or one of his staff by telephoning 020 7911 7127. Inquiries about family proceedings should be addressed to the Team Manager, Family Litigation.

The Official Solicitor's address is:
81 Chancery Lane
London WC2A 1DD
DX 0012 London Chancery Lane
Tel: 020 7911 7127
Fax: 020 7911 7105
Email: enquiries@offsol.gsi.gov.uk

2 April 2001
Laurence Oates, Official Solicitor

Appendix E

Medical certificate for the Official Solicitor with guidance notes

[Ref:]

CERTIFICATE
MENTAL CAPACITY TO MANAGE PROPERTY AND AFFAIRS

Name of patient...

Please read the attached notes before completing this form.

Please answer all questions as fully as you can.

INSTRUCTIONS Insert your full name and address	I .... of ....
Give your medical qualifications	....
	hereby certify as follows:
For a definition of "mental disorder" see note 2 attached	1. I last examined the patient on .... and in my opinion the patient is – *capable of managing and administering his/her* property and affairs *incapable of managing and administering his/her property and affairs by reason of mental disorder,

as defined by section 1(2) of the Mental Health Act 1983.

(*delete as appropriate*)

If in your opinion the Patient is **incapable** of managing his/her property and affairs, please answer questions 2–8.

Your attention is drawn to notes 4 and 5 attached

2. My opinion is based on the following diagnosis and evidence of incapacity –

3. The present mental disorder has lasted since ....

4. The patient's date of birth is ....

5. The patient's prospects of recovery of capacity (whether or not coupled with complete mental recovery) are –

6. Is the patient capable of discussion with my representative or with a solicitor instructed by me concerning legal proceedings?

    ☐YES   ☐NO

    Please comment

7. If so, is such discussion likely to affect him/her detrimentally and if so, in what way?

    ☐YES   ☐NO

    Please comment

8. Any additional comments

    Signed ....

    Dated ....

GUIDANCE NOTES

Please read these notes before completing the Medical Certificate

These notes have been prepared in consultation with The Royal College of Psychiatrists, the British Medical Association and the Court of Protection.

1. Doctors should be aware that if a person who is involved in legal proceedings becomes incapable of managing his property and affairs by reason of mental disorder, his interests must be protected by the appointment of a *next friend* (if he is a plaintiff) or a *guardian ad litem* (if he is a defendant), who will conduct the proceedings on his behalf. The Official Solicitor is usually approached in cases where there is no other suitable person who is willing to act.

2. Before a next friend or guardian ad litem can be appointed, medical evidence must be obtained to establish whether the person is incapable of managing his own property and affairs by reason of mental disorder, as defined in the Mental Health Act 1983. Section 1 (2) of the Act defines mental disorder as:

   "... mental illness, arrested or incomplete development of the mind, psychopathic disorder and any other disorder or disability of mind."

   and psychopathic disorder is defined as:

   "... a persistent disorder or disability of the mind (whether or not including significant impairment of intelligence) which results in abnormally aggressive or seriously irresponsible conduct on the part of the person concerned."

3. Criteria for assessing incapacity are not identical with those for assessing the need for compulsory admission to hospital. The fact that a person is suffering from mental disorder within the meaning of the Mental Health Act 1983, whether living in the community or resident in hospital, detained or informally is not of itself evidence of incapacity to manage his affairs. On the other hand, a person may be so incapable and yet may not be liable for compulsory admission to hospital.

4. The Official Solicitor's certificate requires the doctor to state in paragraph 2 the grounds on which he bases his opinion of incapacity. It is this part of the certificate which most commonly appears to give rise to the most difficulty for the doctor. What is required is a simple statement giving clear evidence of incapacity which an intelligent lay person can understand, eg reference to defect of short term memory, of spatial or temporal orientation or of reasoning ability, or to reckless behaviour (sometimes periodic as in mania) without regard to the future, or evidence of vulnerability to exploitation, or to delusions.

5. In many cases, eg senile dementia, severe brain damage, acute or chronic psychiatric disorder and severe mental impairment the assessment of incapacity may present little difficulty. Cases of functional or personality disorders may give more problems and assessment may depend on the individual doctor's interpretation of mental disorder. It may assist the doctor to know that, particularly in cases of periodic remission, the Official Solicitor will ensure that the patient's condition is regularly reassessed for the purpose of the legal proceedings. In an appropriate case the Official Solicitor will take immediate steps for his removal as guardian ad litem or next friend to enable the patient to resume personal control of his affairs.

Appendix F

Medical certificate for the Court of Protection with notes for guidance

CONFIDENTIAL   *Ref (office use only)-*

COURT OF PROTECTION

MEDICAL CERTIFICATE (CP3)

- Important – please read the attached guidance notes before completing the form
- As this is an official Court document, please ensure that this form is typed if your handwriting is unclear
- If you have any queries about this form, please call our Customer Services helpline: ☎ 0845 330 2900

IN THE MATTER OF

(please use BLOCK CAPITALS)

Full name of patient: ....

Address of patient: ....

....

Post code: ....

Telephone number and date of birth of patient: ☎...................... d.o.b ....

Male/Female (please circle)

Your name: I ....

Your address: of ....

....

Post code: ....

Your telephone number
and e-mail address: ☎.......................... e-mail ....

Your medical
qualifications: ....

declare as follows:

1. I am the medical practitioner for the above-named
   patient and have so acted since: ....

1. I last examined the patient on: ....

   and in my opinion the patient is incapable by reason of
   mental disorder of managing and administering his/her
   property and affairs. (*For a definition of "mental disorder"
   please see note 2 attached*)

2. My opinion is based on the following **diagnosis:** (*Please
   refer to notes 5, 6 and 7 attached*)

   My diagnosis is based on the following **evidence
   of mental incapacity:**

3. The present mental disorder has lasted since: ....
   ....

4. Is the patient a danger to himself/herself
   and/or others in any way?   ☐ Yes ☐ No
   If **yes**, please comment:

5. Does the patient need anything at
   present to provide additional support?   ☐ Yes ☐ No
   If **yes**, what recommendations do
   you make?

6. What is the patient's life expectancy?
    (*Please refer to note 8 attached*) □Under 5 years
                                          □Over 5 years

    Please comment:

---

7. Please give a brief summary of the patient's physical
    condition.

---

8. In your opinion, how capable
    is the patient of appreciating
    his/her surroundings?   □ Capable
                                         □ Limited
                                           capability
    please comment: □ Not capable

---

9. Has the patient made you aware of any   □ Yes □No
    views he/she has about his/her future
    care and welfare?

    If **yes**, please comment:

---

10. Do you consider that in respect of this   □ Yes □No

    patient there is a prospect of a recovery
    in the patient's mental capacity?
    (*Please refer to note 9 attached*)

    If **no**, please state the reasons why:

    If **yes**, please state:
    a. Why you consider that there is a prospect of mental
        recovery in this case.

    b. When the Court might usefully enquire further to
        establish whether or not the patient has demonstrated
        a sufficient level of mental recovery to be able to
        manage and administer his/her property and affairs.

11.	Is the patient capable of understanding that an application is being made to appoint a receiver to manage and administer his/her property and affairs?	☐ Yes ☐ No
	Please comment:	

12.	Do you consider that the patient should receive verbal notice of the application to appoint a receiver? (*Please refer to note 10 attached*)	☐ Yes ☐ No
	If **yes**, please indicate who you consider to be the best person to give such notice and comment further below	☐Close relative or friend ☐Professional carer ☐Social Worker ☐Medical Practitioner ☐Legal Representative ☐Psychiatrist ☐Other (please specify)

13.	Have you or your family or friends any financial interest in the accommodation in which the patient is living or in any other matter concerning the patient?	☐Yes ☐No
	If **yes**, please give details:	

---

14. General comments and any other
    recommendations for future care:

I declare that to the best of my knowledge and belief,the
information I have given on this form is true and accurate:

Signature: ....

Name (print): .... **Date:** ....

NOTES FOR GUIDANCE

- **Please read these notes before completing the Medical Certificate.**
- **Please note that when the Medical Certificate has been completed its contents will be confidential to the Court and those authorised by the Court to see it.**
- **These notes have been prepared in consultation with the British Medical Association. The BMA sets the level of fees and reviews the fees on an annual basis.**

1. Doctors should be aware that if a person owning real or personal property becomes incapable, by reason of mental disorder, of safeguarding and managing his affairs, an application should be made to the Court of Protection for the appointment of a receiver for such directions as may be necessary.

2. An application to the Court of Protection for the appointment of a receiver for directions must be supported by a medical certificate stating that, in the doctor's opinion, the patient is incapable of managing and administering his property and affairs by reason of mental disorder as defined in Section 1 of the Mental Health Act 1983. "Mental Disorder" is defined in Section 1(2) of the act as meaning "mental illness, arrested or incomplete development of mind, psychopathic disorder and any other disorder or disability of mind", and "psychopathic disorder" is defined as "persistent disorder

or disability of the mind (whether or not including significant impairment of intelligence) which results in abnormally aggressive or seriously irresponsible conduct on the part of the person concerned".

3.   Criteria for assessing incapacity are not identical with those for assessing the need for compulsory admission to hospital. The fact that a person is suffering from mental disorder within the meaning of the Mental Health Act 1983, whether living in the community or resident in hospital, detained or informal, is not of itself evidence of incapacity to manage his affairs. On the other hand, a person may be so incapable and yet not be liable to compulsory admission to hospital.

4.   The certifying doctor may be either the person's general practitioner or any other registered medical practitioner who has examined the patient.

5.   The Medical Certificate requires the doctor to state in paragraph 3 the nature of the mental disorder and the grounds on which he/she bases his opinion of incapacity. What is required is a diagnosis and a statement giving clear evidence of incapacity, for example, reference to defect of short-term memory, of spatial and temporal orientation or of reasoning ability, or to reckless spending (sometimes periodic as in mania) without regard for the future, or evidence of vulnerability to exploitation. It is especially important that the evidence of incapacity shows how the incapacity prevents the patient from being able to administer and manage his/her financial affairs.

6.   In many cases of senile dementia, severe brain damage, acute or chronic psychiatric disorder and severe mental impairment the assessment of incapacity should present little difficulty. Cases of functional and personality disorders may give more problems and assessment may depend on the individual doctor's interpretation of mental disorder. The Court tends toward the view that these conditions may render a person liable to the Court's jurisdiction where there appears to be a real danger that the disorder will lead to dissipation of considerable capital assets.

7. A person may not be dealt with under the Mental Health Act 1983, and may not be the subject of an application to the Court of Protection by reason only of promiscuity or other immoral conduct, sexual deviancy or dependence on alcohol or drugs.

8. In Paragraph 7, the information you are asked to provide on life expectancy is useful in that it helps the Court to determine an appropriate investment policy for the patient.

9. The Court recongnises that it is difficult for general practitioners or consultant psychiatrists to specify whether there is a prospect of a recovery in the patient's mental capacity in a particular case. However, under the Human Rights Act 1998, the Court is under a proactive obligation to find out if a patient will be fit to resume management of his/her own affairs. It would therefore assist the Court if you could indicate whether the patient is likely to demonstrate a sufficient level of recovery to be able to manage and administer his/her own property and affairs.

10. In all cases, the patient must be given formal notice of any application to the Court of Protection for a receiver to be appointed on his/her behalf. This is in order to comply with the European Convention on Human Rights and the Human Rights Act 1998. Notification provides the patient with the opportunity to express views about the appointment of a particular person or contribute other information, which will assist the Court in reaching a decision. Normally, notice of any application is given by personally serving a letter on the patient. The Court however recognises that some patients will not be in a position to comprehend the notice that is given to them. For some patients it may therefore be better if a relative, friend or professional person such as a carer, social worker, legal representative or medical practitioner explained the notice verbally to them. It may also be preferable for the notice to be given verbally because of the risk to the patient's health or distress that might be caused to the patient by receipt of a written notice on its own. It would therefore be helpful to the Court if you could indicate whether in this case notice should be

explained verbally and who would be the best person to give such notice.

The completed Medical Certificate should be returned to either the solicitors acting in the matter or to:

Public Guardianship Office
Archway Tower
2 Junction Road
London
N19 5SZ

Data Protection Act 1998

The Court of Protection (an office of the Supreme Court) exists to protect the property and financial affairs of persons suffering from mental disorders. The Public Guardianship Office carries out the day-to-day administrative functions of the Court. Information that you provide in these forms will be retained and used initially by the Court to determine how the property and financial affairs of the incapacitated person will be managed & administered.

COURT OF PROTECTION

> THE INFORMATION CONTAINED IN THIS FORM IS CONFIDENTIAL AND MUST NOT BE DISCLOSED TO ANY OTHER PARTY UNLESS THE COURT SO DIRECTS

IN THE MATTER OF

MEDICAL CERTIFICATE - CP3

Appendix G

Sample letter: Test of capacity

The test of capacity depends on the subject area. This example uses testamentary capacity. Different tests apply to, for example, capacity to litigate. Please refer to the relevant chapter for the specific test.

Dear Dr [...]

Re: Client's name [X] date of birth [...] and solicitor's reference [...]

I am instructed on behalf of [X] who wishes me to prepare a will on his/her behalf. As you may be aware, the law requires wills that are drawn up for an elderly person or for someone who is seriously ill to be witnessed or approved by a medical practitioner. In accordance with good practice I am therefore writing to request that you assess [X's] capacity to make a will and prepare a report which may be used in evidence in the event that there is any subsequent legal challenge.

I attach evidence of [X's] consent for you to disclose medical information for the purpose of this report.

You may wish to note that you need only show on the balance of probability whether [X] has or does not have testamentary capacity, in other words, that it is more likely than not. I also request that you pay particular attention to the following points, and indicate whether [X] understands them.

- The nature of the act of making a will. This involves understanding that s/he will die and that when s/he does the will comes into operation. Further, s/he can change or revoke the will before his/her death, but only for as long as s/he has the mental capacity to do so.
- The effect of making a will. This includes the appointment of executors, deciding who receives what, whether the gifts are outright, the consequences of a depleted estate, that a beneficiary may pre-decease him/her, and the effect on any previous will.
- The extent of the estate. This includes the amount of property or money or investments s/he holds and the fact that some may be

jointly owned, that some benefits may be payable only on his/her death irrespective of his/her will, and that the estate may change during his/her lifetime.

- The possible claims of others. Beneficiaries may be left out because of other adequate provision, or because of personal reasons. [X] must be aware of these reasons and the possibility that these could be challenged.

I attach details of [X]'s estate for your reference along with a draft will which s/he has agreed to disclose.

As you may be aware, a diagnosis of mental disorder does not necessarily mean that [X] lacks capacity. It would be helpful therefore to include in your report details of any abnormality or disability of mental state. I would be grateful if you would also include reference to [X]'s physical state in so far as it is relevant to this report.

I have requested you prepare this report because [X] informs me that you have been his/her family doctor for a number of years. If, however, in the course of taking a psychiatric history and conducting a mental state examination you consider a specialist report is required (for example from a psychiatrist or psychologist), please let me know.

I confirm that we have agreed the sum of £ ... ... for the purposes of the examination and preparation of this report. In the unlikely event that you are required to give evidence at court a further fee will be negotiated. Please mark your invoice with the reference stated at the top of this letter.

If you require any further information or clarification on any points please do not hesitate to contact me.

Yours sincerely

Useful addresses

The British Medical Association

BMA House
Tavistock Square
London WC1H 9JP
Tel: 020 7387 4499
Medical ethics: 020 7383 6286
http://www.bma.org.uk

The Law Society

113 Chancery Lane
London WC2A 1PL
DX 56 London/Chancery Lane
Tel: 020 7242 1222
Mental Health & Disability Committee: 020 7320 5695
Lawyer line advice and information: 0870 606 2588
http://www.lawsociety.org.uk

Official addresses

Court of Protection
  Archway Tower
  2 Junction Road
  London N19 5SZ
  DX 141150 Archway 2
  Tel: 020 7664 7178

Official Solicitor and Public Trustee
  81 Chancery Lane
  London WC2A 1DD
  DX 0012 London/Chancery Lane
  Tel: 020 7911 7127
  http://www.offsol.demon.co.uk

Principal Registry of the Family Division
First Avenue House
42–46 High Holborn
London WC1V 6NP
DX 396 London/Chancery Lane
Tel: 020 7947 6000

Public Guardianship Office
Archway Tower
2 Junction Road
London N19 5SZ
DX 141150 Archway 2
Tel: 0845 330 2900
http://www.guardianship.gov.uk

Royal Courts of Justice
Strand
London WC1A 2LL
DX 396 London/Chancery Lane
Tel: 020 7947 6000
(In emergencies, an RCJ Security Officer will contact lawyers
from the Official Solicitor's Office)

Treasury Solicitor
Queen Anne's Chambers
28 Broadway
London SW1H 9JX
DX 123242 St James's Park
Tel: 020 7210 3000
http://www.treasury-solicitor.gov.uk

General

Age Concern Cymru (Wales)
Fourth Floor
1 Cathedral Road
Cardiff CF11 9SD
Tel: 029 2037 1566
http://www.accymru.org.uk

Age Concern England
  Astral House
  1268 London Road
  London SW16 4ER
  Tel: 020 8679 8000
  Information line: 0800 009966
  http://www.ageconcern.org.uk

Action on Elder Abuse
  Astral House
  1268 London Road
  London SW16 4ER
  Helpline: 0880 8808 8042
  http://www.elderabuse.org.uk

Alzheimer's Society
  Gordon House
  10 Greencoat Place
  London SW1P 1PH
  Helpline: 0845 300 0336
  http://www.alzheimers.org.uk

Carers UK
  Ruth Pitter House
  20–25 Glasshouse Yard
  London EC1A 1JS
  Tel: 020 7490 8824
  Carers line: 0808 808 7777
  http://www.carersonline.org.uk

Counsel and Care for the Elderly
  Twyman House
  16 Bonny Street
  London NW1 9PG
  Helpline: 0845 300 7585
  http://www.counselandcare.org.uk

Down's Syndrome Association
  153–155 Mitcham Road
  London SW17 9PG
  Tel: 020 8682 4001
  http://www.downs-syndrome.org.uk

Headway (Brain Injuries Association)
  4 King Edward Court
  King Edward Street
  Nottingham NG1 1EW
  Helpline: 0808 800 2244
  http://www.headway.org.uk

Help the Aged
  16–18 St James's Walk
  Clerkenwell Green
  London EC1R 0BE
  Advice line: 0808 800 6565
  http://www.helptheaged.org.uk

MIND (National Association for Mental Health)
  15–19 Broadway
  London E15 4BQ
  Tel: 020 8519 2122
  Information line: 08457 660 163
  http://www.mind.org.uk

Mencap (Royal Society for Mentally Handicapped Children and Adults)
  123 Golden Lane
  London EC1Y 0RT
  Tel: 020 7454 0454
  Helpline: 0808 808 1111
  http://www.mencap.org.uk

National Autistic Society
  393 City Road
  London EC1V 1NG
  Tel: 020 7833 2299
  Helpline: 0870 600 8585
  http://www.nas.org.uk

Patients Association
  PO Box 935
  Harrow
  Middlesex HA1 3YJ
  Tel: 020 8423 9119
  Helpline: 0845 608 4455
  http://www.patients-association.com

SANE
First Floor
Cityside House
40 Alder Street
London E1 1EE
Helpline: 0845 767 8000
http://www.sane.org.uk

Stroke Association
Stroke House
240 City Road
London EC1V 2PR
Tel: 020 7566 0300
Helpline: 0845 3033 1000
http://www.stroke.org.uk

VOICE UK
PO Box 238
Derby DE1 9NJ
Tel: 0870 013 3965
http://www.voiceuk.clara.net

Further reading

Law Society publications

Ashton GR, Edis A. *Elderly client handbook, 3rd ed*. London: The Law Society, 2004.

The Law Society. *The guide to the professional conduct of solicitors, 8th ed*. London: The Law Society, 1999.

Postgate D, Taylor C. *Advising mentally disordered offenders*. London: The Law Society, 2000.

Law Society guidance is available on line at http://www.lawsociety.org.uk.

British Medical Association publications

British Medical Association. *Advance statements about medical treatment*. London: BMA, 1995.

British Medical Association. *The older person: consent and care*. London: BMA, 1995.

British Medical Association. *Medical ethics today: the BMA's handbook of ethics and law, 2nd ed*. London: BMJ Books, 2004.

British Medical Association. *Withholding and withdrawing life-prolonging medical treatment: guidance for decision making, 2nd ed*. London: BMJ Books, 2001.

Many BMA publications and guidance are available on line at http://www.bma.org.uk/ethics.

Law Commission publications

Law Commission. *Mentally incapacitated adults and decision-making: an overview*. London: HMSO, 1991 (Law Com No 119).

Law Commission. *Mentally incapacitated adults and decision-making: a new jurisdiction*. London: HMSO, 1993 (Law Com No 128).

Law Commission. *Mentally incapacitated adults and decision-making: medical treatment and research*. London: HMSO, 1993 (Law Com No 129).

Law Commission. *Mentally incapacitated adults and other vulnerable adults: public law protection*. London: HMSO, 1993 (Law Com No 130).

Law Commission. *Mental incapacity*. London: HMSO, 1995 (Law Com No 231).

Other relevant publications

Law relating to mental incapacity

Ashton GR, ed. *Butterworths older client law service.* London: Butterworths Tolley, 1997 (looseleaf).

Ashton GR. *Elderly people and the law.* London: Butterworths, 1995.

Ashton GR. *Mental handicap and the law.* London: Sweet & Maxwell, 1992.

Bartlett P, Sandland R. *Mental health law: policy and practice.* London: Blackstone Press, 2000.

Department of Health, Welsh Office. *Mental Health Act code of practice.* London: The Stationery Office, 1999.

Jones R. *Mental Health Act manual, 8th ed.* London: Sweet & Maxwell, 2003.

Lush D. *Elderly clients: a precedent manual.* Bristol: Jordans, 1996.

Whitehouse C, ed. *Finance and law for the older client.* London: Butterworths Tolley, 2000 (looseleaf).

Medical treatment

Harper RS. *Medical treatment and the law: the protection of adults and minors in the Family Division.* Bristol: Family Law, 1999.

Kennedy I, Grubb A. *Medical law: text with materials, 3rd ed.* London: Butterworths, 2000.

Mason JK, McCall Smith RA, Laurie GT. *Law and medical ethics, 6th ed.* Edinburgh: Butterworths, 2002.

Silberfeld M, Fish A. *When the mind fails: a guide to dealing with incompetency.* Toronto: University Press, 1994.

Financial management

Kenny P, Kenny A. *Powers of attorney: the new law.* Newcastle: Northumbria Law Press, 2000.

Lush D. *Cretney and Lush on enduring powers of attorney, 5th ed.* Bristol: Jordans, 2001.

Lush D, ed. *Heyward and Massey: Court of Protection practice, 13th ed.* London: Sweet and Maxwell, 2002 (looseleaf).

Terrell M. *A practitioner's guide to the Court of Protection.* London: Butterworths Tolley, 2002.

Inheritance

Wright CE, ed. *Butterworths wills, probate and administration services.* London: Butterworths Tolley, 1996 (looseleaf).

Index

Page numbers in **bold** type refer to figures; those in *italic* refer to boxed material.

As the subject of this book is mental capacity and its assessment, entries under these terms have been kept to a minimum. Readers are advised to consult more specific entries. Mental capacity has been referred to as capacity throughout.